Taller, Slimmer, Younger

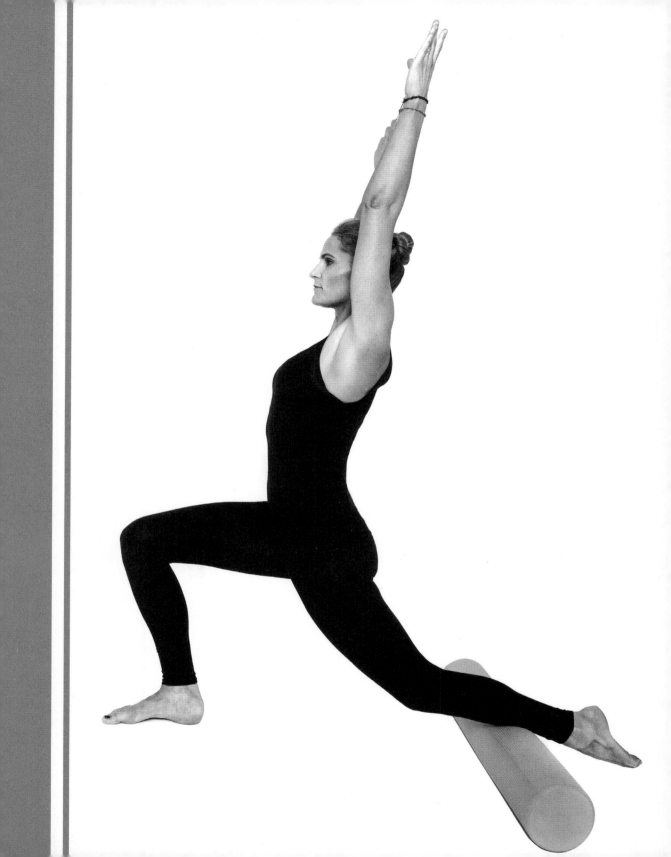

Taller, Slimmer, Younger

21 Days to a Foam Roller Physique

LAUREN ROXBURGH

Vermilion
LONDON

10 9 8 7 6 5 4 3 2 1

Vermilion, an imprint of Ebury Publishing,
20 Vauxhall Bridge Road,
London SW1V 2SA

Vermilion is part of the Penguin Random House group of companies
whose addresses can be found at global.penguinrandomhouse.com

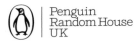
Penguin
Random House
UK

First published in the United Kingdom by Vermilion in 2016
First published in the United States by Ballantine Books, an imprint
of Random House, a division of Penguin Random House LLC, New York in 2016

Book design by Mary A. Wirth

www.eburypublishing.co.uk

A CIP catalogue record for this book is available from the British Library

ISBN 9781785040580

Printed and bound in China by C&C Offset Printing Co., Ltd

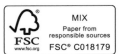

Penguin Random House is committed to a sustainable
future for our business, our readers and our planet.
This book is made from Forest Stewardship Council®
certified paper.

*Bursting with love
to Gus and Cameron Roxburgh,
for believing in me*

Contents

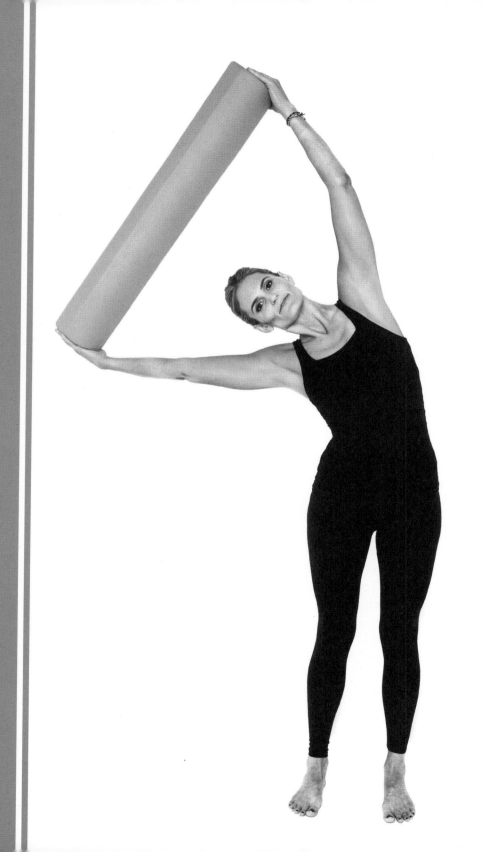

Introduction

Align Your Body, Align Your Life

When the body gets working appropriately,
the force of gravity can flow through. Then,
spontaneously, the body heals itself.

—IDA P. ROLF, PHD

When I met my client and now dear friend Kristen in 2009, she was working out really hard with a trainer three to five times a week. Her body was thick, bulky, tired, heavy, sore, and constantly riddled with pain. I told her about the 10-minute-per-day foam rolling program I had designed and how it had completely transformed my body. I told her I could do the same thing for her, but that I needed her to trust in me, even though a few of the things I would ask her to do might feel scary. Kristen's initial response was skeptical. "Oh, you're just naturally skinny. I will never have that body," she scoffed. I responded by showing Kristen pictures of my larger self. She was blown away by the difference and agreed to give my program a shot. Sure enough, after a few weeks on the program, Kristen lost three inches in her hips, simply from releasing the toxins that were stored in her fascia and reducing the bulkiness in her dense muscles. She went from a size 30 jeans to a size 26 without starving herself. And the pain? Totally gone.

I understand all of the frustration and fear Kristen felt about getting in shape because I've been there. Although I've worked with hundreds of clients, I am first and foremost my own guinea pig. I've been a swimmer since the age of four. As a collegiate athlete and water polo player, I pushed myself constantly, yet still wasn't satisfied with what I saw in the mirror. I read all of the fitness magazines and books, and they all recited the same mantra over and over again: *Run more! Do more cardio! Eat like a bird!* So I did. The end result was that I had great muscle tone, but was also hungry, thick, very stiff and tense, and generally far from feeling like my best self. It wasn't until I ditched the cardio and intense training and turned to relieving, aligning, stretching, and toning my body with the foam roller that things began to change in a big way. Suddenly, I was taller, slimmer, and looked and felt younger. My pain diminished and I felt so much calmer. My body became more streamlined and lithe. The muscles I had overworked relaxed, and my intrinsic (or "ballerina") muscles started revealing themselves. Best of all, I *felt* better. It's safe to say that I look way better at thirty-seven than I ever did in my twenties. And, might I add, this program allowed me to maintain all of this post-pregnancy.

Kristen and I are not alone in our results. Over the course of the past fifteen years, I have applied this same program to everyone from top pro athletes to celebrities to everyday people of all shapes and sizes. Across the board, everyone who has completed my foam rolling program has undergone a complete transformation not only physically but also mentally and emotionally. Even more than seeing clients who transform their physique, I love to watch clients use this program as a means of combating and resolving chronic pain. It's like giving someone the gift of freedom.

I know it sounds like hocus-pocus that ten minutes per day of foam rolling can lead to such transformative results, but there's actually a proven science to the program I've designed. The foam roller works in a way that nothing else on the market right now does because it targets a newly discovered organ: fascia, or connective tissue. We're ultimately working with the fascia on the foam roller, and that's why this technique is so innovative. We'll delve into what fascia is and why it matters in the next chapter, but for now, suffice it to say that the science and medical communities really only came to discover fascia and its role in our physiology in the past decade—2006, to be exact. Working with fascia is still a revolutionary, cutting-edge approach to fitness, as it essentially offers a means to simply and effectively reshape the body.

I first discovered the roller more than fifteen years ago when I was working as a personal trainer at a health club in Manhattan Beach, California. As many trainers and physical therapists do, I learned how to use the roller for self-massage. I immediately loved this technique and used it with my clients from day one to warm them up before their workout program. Fast-forward to my first Pilates workshop a few years later, and I was reintroduced to the roller as a tool for mimicking many of the elongating and core-strengthening moves traditionally performed on expensive Pilates equipment. This was a breakthrough moment for me because it allowed me to empower my clients, whenever and wherever they were, with an easy way of consistently performing the Pilates moves. I couldn't help but notice that once my Pilates clients began incorporating the roller into their routine, their bodies transformed more rapidly. A few years later, I went to school for Structural Integration and learned so much more about the body, fascia, and the anatomy of movement. This knowledge allowed me to take rolling to an entirely new level, and formed the basis of the program you're about to embark on over the course of the next twenty-one days.

Only recently have the medical and fitness worlds discovered a little secret that I've understood for a long time now—that the foam roller is good for so much more than aiding in physical therapy or just working out knots and tightness. When used regularly and correctly, it can be utterly transformative and unbelievably healing. My revolutionary foam rolling program combines lengthening and toning Pilates-based exercises with self-care movements that dig into the body's connective tissues, thus reshaping the musculature and the actual structure of the body and releasing those toxins and blockages that wreak so much havoc. The result of this is a real, healthy, balanced body that's nurtured, loved, strong, and appreciated. Through this program you will discover the most elongated, relaxed, femininely toned, uniformly developed, and joyful version of you. You'll understand how freeing it feels to have a body that's aligned (lots more to come about how and why this is so important) and a sense of yourself that's ageless and draws you into a place where your soul can really soar. The real magic bullet to this plan is that it will make you feel *fantastic* about yourself and develop in you a vibrancy you probably didn't even know was possible. And once you get to that place ... well, anything is possible!

Another critical difference between the program you're about to embark on and the others you've probably tried before is that this one is all about taking care of yourself rather than being a slave to working out. It's about taking a holistic, healthy approach to fitness and wellness and doing so in a manner that actually feels good. Yes, you will get fit in the process, but you will also deepen your mind-body connection and learn to really listen, inhabit, and care for your body.

Self-care may sound indulgent, but the fact is that it's never been more important than it is today. The fast-paced globalized world we live in has a tendency to make us feel like we need to be in three places at once, doing three things all at the same time. "*Go, go, go!*" our system screams at us. As a result, our fight-or-flight response is constantly switched on, which means we're in the midst of a constant adrenaline surge; our bodies are chronically compressed from the stress and tension of it all, which slows down our restorative systems. Obviously, technology is not going away any time soon, so it's increasingly imperative that we take the time to unplug, tune in to our bodies, and give ourselves a bit of self-care, which will ultimately help us become more efficient and clear-headed. This is the only way to prevent the type of hunched-over, shorter, tense, wider, thicker, defeated body that the modern world breeds. My program will start reversing that process right now.

So much of our physical state is a result of the stress and tension we carry around on a day-to-day basi s. When we're stressed, we store up toxins and our energy (or *chi*, an Eastern concept that translates to life force) gets blocked. We become physically, mentally, and emotionally stagnant and our systems slow down. Lugging emotions, trauma, guilt, resentment, and memories with us can age us, wreak havoc on our bodies and health, and result in a host of serious long-term consequences, such as excess weight, anxiety, pain, anger, and even a reduction in height. Minimizing stress helps fire up our bodies by regulating stress hormones and jump-starting our metabolism.

Over the course of the many years I've spent working as a certified Pilates instructor, Structural Integration specialist and personal trainer, one of the most important lessons I've learned is that the body works as a whole. No matter how much you want great abs or slim thighs (both of which you *can* have, by the way), falling into a stale routine that focuses on just one thing really doesn't work. It's not healthy; in fact, it throws your body completely out of alignment. Our bodies are designed to move fluidly in all directions, and targeted exercises simply don't allow for this natural movement. When you move away from stagnation and repetition, get back to your natural movement patterns, and release stress through your breath and flowing body, you become more balanced in your musculature and in how you carry weight. Moreover, you will tune in to yourself and the world around you, and will be more full of life, joy, and energy. This is not to mention the excess weight that melts off as if by magic when we get back to moving as we are meant to. By the time you're finished with this program, you'll be back in touch with those natural movement patterns, which is life-changing in and of itself.

Obtaining true well-being and a stunning physique involves working with the body as a whole, three-dimensionally, from top to bottom *and* from the inside out. A healthy, productive, mindful routine will do more than make you feel physically better; it will also enhance you mentally and emotionally, and help you make healthier diet and lifestyle choices. In fact, for many of my clients, regardless of the physical reasons that led them to me in the first place, it's the emotional and mental benefits they receive from my program that propel them to adopt a regular, consistent routine and keep them coming back for more. It's a joke among my clients that they know who works with Lo (as they call me)—they can see it in their eyes and, of course, in their bodies. That inner and outer glow, hot body, zest for life, and extra spunk in their step is always a giveaway.

But it's okay to start with the simple goal of being more fit. It's where most of us start. And this 21-day program *will* produce the physical results you're looking for ... and then some. You'll gain streamlined definition, a new glow, and a calmer, more relaxed vibe; and you will walk taller and with more confidence than you ever have before. More than that, the program I'll share in this book will connect you with your body, eliminate chronic issues, and help build new and healthy habits. *And* I've saved the best part for last: This 21-day program isn't a punishing, unsustainable workout regimen. In fact, I like to think of it as the anti-workout workout. As you feel the stress and tension melting away and your body lengthening and leaning out, I bet you'll actually come to look forward to your daily rolling sessions!

Taller, Slimmer, Younger

The TSY 21-Day Program

How and Why It Works

Let's talk about what it means to be taller, slimmer, and younger (or, as I like to call it, TSY). A TSY body is not an obsessive, starved, overworked, or superficial body. It's not the type of body that you torture yourself to obtain only to find that if you *do* achieve the results you're looking for in the first place, they're logistically impossible to maintain over time. Our body naturally wants to *thrive*, and indeed it does when it is loved by the person who is inhabiting it.

We've been told for so long that in order to look and feel good, we *have* to burn calories, push ourselves to the limit, and restrict our diets to the point where there's no real pleasure in eating. I am delighted to tell you that this is simply *not true*! My years of experience working with clients from all walks of life have proven this time and time again.

Over the next twenty-one days, you will essentially be using the foam roller to regenerate soft tissue and elongate and sculpt the right muscles in the most balanced and healthy way, as well as relaxing the ones that need a break. I'll also teach you how to work smarter, not harder, and give you tips to employ while you are moving through your normal day, walking from Point A to Point B. I'll show you simple things you can do daily to take better care of yourself mentally and emotionally, and to transform yourself from the inside out.

To accomplish this, you'll learn how to use the roller for a couple of different purposes. Each day of rolling includes two different movement categories: Smooth-out and Reshape. You will begin each day focusing on a particular section of the body and using the roller to melt down and hydrate the fascia and connective tissue, thus releasing toxins, inflammation, thickness, stiffness, and density; getting rid of scar tissue; and generally clearing out blockages in your body. Essentially, throughout the program you'll be giving yourself a full-scale bodywork session and waking up all the muscles that make you long, lean, and glowing. Those of you who experience chronic tension and pain will be astounded at what a release these movements offer. Once we've created that "fresh slate," we'll move on to the Reshape movements. This is where we will tone and elongate muscles with Pilates-based core exercises that incorporate the roller.

Just as important as working fascia and muscle, this program also incorporates methods for breathing, decreasing stress, and calming the nervous system. When we're nervous and stressed, among other things, we tend not to breathe. Deep, full breathing is *so* important to optimal health. Even though oxygen is a basic necessity of life, we *all* breathe shallowly and/or hold our breath. And we especially do it when we're stressed out. I had a client lose ten pounds over the course of a few weeks just by learning to slow down and breathe more deeply. Breathing calms you down, draws you into the present moment, and makes you far more aware of yourself and the world around you. When you're present and aware, everything changes—the stress eating goes away (especially the sugar cravings), you feel less pressed for time, and you make better choices. You'll be amazed at how much a calmer and more balanced demeanor curbs emotional eating and naturally shifts your diet and overall lifestyle into a healthier state. The cumulative result of all of these changes is that you'll look and feel TSY—taller, slimmer, and younger.

Roll Your Way Taller

Lots of fitness regimens claim that they can make you slimmer and more fit, but I bet you've never heard of one that can make you taller, right? Well, this one can. Believe it or not, I can help you grow an inch to an inch and a half—I've seen it happen, both with myself and with my clients. But perhaps not in the way you're thinking. The rolling sequences in this book naturally lead you toward proper posture—an increasingly foreign state in this world where we're constantly hunching over our desks or tapping away on e-devices.

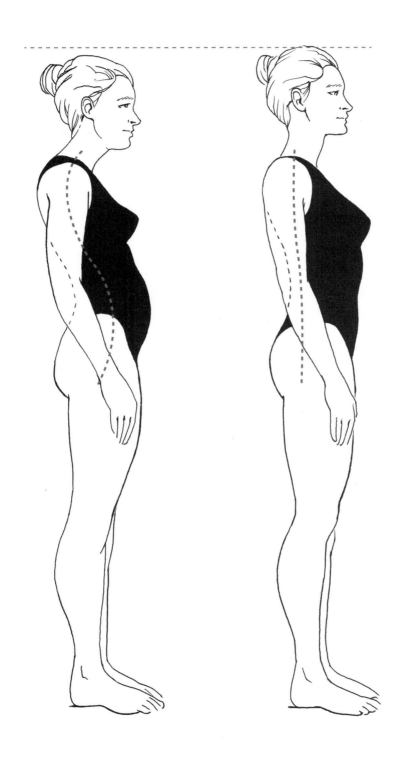

Despite what your grandmother may have told you, good posture isn't about balancing a book on your head. It's about increasing your core strength, and joint decompression which supports the spine and improves its alignment. This is accomplished through a series of exercises that improve posture while decompressing the spine and other joints, thus not only increasing height but also enhancing body awareness. Essentially, being taller is about improving your body's relationship with gravity and the manner in which you present yourself to the world.

Most likely, you are *not* utilizing all of the space you have available in your body; the exercises in this book will ensure that the full amount of space available in the vertebrae and joints is activated, thus increasing height. Even if that increase is measured in millimeters, the effect is huge. It allows you to tap into your body's maximum height and provides a level of freedom that gives the impression of length and confidence. While there's nothing you can do to lengthen bones, these weight-bearing exercises can help strengthen them. Even better, they can help prevent osteoporosis, joint compression, spinal shrinkage, and all of the postural problems that come with these conditions.

You'll walk away from this 21-day program with your head (literally) held higher, your heart open, and the new confidence that comes from standing up tall, claiming your space, and facing the world.

Roll Your Way Slimmer

When I ask my clients what their primary goal is, most of them tell me that they want to slim down. Some people strive for more svelte bellies, while others want to zero in on toning their thighs, arms, or butt. Within this program you'll find solutions for all of those areas that we most want to see leaned out and elongated.

Being slim is about so much more than just being skinny—it's about being strong. That requires toning and elongating the intrinsic and core muscles (or, as I like to call them, the "ballerina muscles"). It's about accessing and connecting to the specific muscles that help pull in the waist, which combats the thickening we all experience as we age. Being slimmer also requires exercises that stimulate the lymphatic system, hydrate the tissues, align and lengthen the body, and flush out toxins. Not only does this aid in weight loss, but it also decreases stress and calms the nervous system, which often results in eating more consciously and less emotionally. Being slimmer is about creating a more toned, calmer, healthier version of you. All of that may sound like a tall order, but you'll be shocked at what a cinch it really is with the pragmatic and consistent application of my program and use of the foam roller.

Unfair as it is, some of us have a body type that seems to get broader and bulkier the more we exercise the way we're told we should (cardio, weight lifting, spinning, boot camp, etc.). I certainly know that was the case for me! The beauty of the foam rolling exercises is that, when done consistently, they will repattern your musculature to adopt that elongated, leaned-out, sculpted look that many of us have given up on as unachievable. Moreover, as you work your fascia with the roller, stored-up toxins will be released, removing bulk and density from your muscles and clearing the way for nice, lean muscle mass. Believe it or not, I've seen people completely thin out certain parts of their body just by rolling out whatever toxins are stuck and activate the proper muscles.

As you roll out the bad stuff, you will also build the esthetically beautiful and equally functionnal muscles. De-bulking muscles that are overworked and overdeveloped will better allow you to turn *on* and connect to the intrinsic stabilizing muscles—the core, the inner thighs, the triceps, and the obliques. Not coincidentally, these are the muscles that tend to fall by the wayside as we age. It's a "use 'em or lose 'em" type of situation; the TSY muscles turn into hanging or lazy muscles when they're not put to use. You'll roll these muscles back into action, rebuilding your connection to and awareness of them. Just ten minutes a day will wake up those neuromuscular connections so that during the many other hours of the day when you're not on the roller—when you're bringing in the groceries, picking the kids up from school, or sitting at your desk—you'll still be aware of your core. Through this awareness, you can keep these core muscles firing and feel more connected to your body. The crazy thing is, after a while you probably won't even be aware that you're doing this. It's all about building healthy new habits.

Roll Your Way Younger

Unfortunately, I can't direct you to the Fountain of Youth. But I can actually share with you something even better: proven tools for living life in such a way that the aging process slows drastically. Combating the effects of aging has everything to do with decreasing stress, releasing tension, and smoothing out scar tissue in order to move more freely. Sounds familiar by this point, right? I will teach you how to do all of this, as well as how to properly hydrate your tissue and lubricate your joints with synovial fluid, thus increasing circulation and reducing tension and rigidity. This will in turn tune you in to your body, allowing you to get to the root of any imbalances, pain, and blockages that may result in premature aging. It may not be the Fountain of Youth ... but it sure as heck is the next best thing!

What You'll Need to Get Started

I'm a firm believer that everyone deserves access to the information necessary to keep them healthy, so when I developed this program, it was important to me that it not be cost prohibitive. This is yet another reason I'm such a fan of the foam roller. This one relatively inexpensive piece of equipment replaces the need for expensive workout equipment, gym or studio membership fees, and costly body-work sessions.

If you don't already have a foam roller on hand, take a look at the box below to help find the option that works best for you. The only additional piece of equipment I recommend is an exercise or yoga mat—whatever you have on hand will do. Essentially, you want to have a surface to work on that simultaneously provides traction and allows you to roll smoothly.

Tips for Purchasing the Right Foam Roller

If you haven't yet armed yourself with a foam roller, now's the time to do so. Foam rollers range from 12 to 35 inches (30 to 90 centimeters) in length. For the purposes of this book, you'll want to use a 35-by-5.75-inch roller. This longer size will allow you to use your roller as a toning tool and will ensure that you can place it perpendicular to your spine for full support and proper alignment.

Foam rollers come in a range of densities. The type of roller you want to use for this program is very specific. Think of yourself as Goldilocks when it comes to selecting the right one: A roller that is too soft won't effectively sculpt and tone fascia and muscle; a roller that is too dense will be too aggressive for the restorative and calming sequences in this program. You want a versatile roller that will give you just the right balance between shaping and restoring. You also want a roller that is durable and that won't break down with regular use. Rollers aren't particularly expensive, but spending an extra ten dollars to begin with will ensure that you're investing in a roller that will last, as opposed to purchasing one that will need to be replaced in a few months' time.

I've spent the past few years testing out rollers of all densities, compos-itions, sizes, and brands. After failing to identify a roller that served all of my and my clients' needs, I decided to take matters into my own hands and develop a line of multifunctional rollers designed to cater to the goals of this program. My line is called Lauren Roxburgh Rollers and can be found on my website at laurenroxburgh .com. These rollers are that perfect medium density that works both for sculpting and for restoration. They are highly durable without being too aggressive, and the textured surface has been specially designed for the multifunctional use of clearing blockages and stimulating the lymphatic system. In simple terms, this means they will help reduce cellulite and bloating, not to mention bolstering immunity.

In a perfect world, I would recommend that everyone have two foam rollers of different sizes. A travel one (12 by 6 inches) to throw in your carry-on bag and use when you're on the fly in your hotel room to help maintain alignment; and a 35-by-5.75-inch roller when doing your daily program.

The 10 Series

The path we'll follow to get to this TSY body is the 10 Series. Over the course of the next twenty-one days, we'll thoroughly target ten different areas of the body. These target areas are based on the systematic "recipe" of the 10 Series of Struc-tural Integration (more about this on page 15), with additional Pilates-based move-ments incorporated to create and enhance muscle tone, strength, and alignment. The ten areas we'll focus on are:

1. Chest, Shoulders and Arms
2. Feet, Ankles, and Lower Legs
3. Legs
4. Waist
5. Tush

6. Hips
7. Pelvis and Inner Thighs
8. Deep Core and Psoas
9. Back of the Core
10. Collarbone, Neck, and Jaw

Over the course of the next twenty-one days, you'll run through the 10 Series twice, leaving a Restorative Day for rest and self-care in the middle. Although all of these exercises inherently merge together mind and body, we'll focus a bit more on the physicality of our work during the first ten days and then draw our attention to the emotional component of it all for the second series of ten. I should also mention here that although we'll focus on certain areas of the body each day, in actuality, all of these exercises target the *entire* body and result in a full-body workout. It all boils down to a matter of emphasis.

The time frame and breakdown of this program are not incidental. Ancient wisdom from many cultures holds that it takes approximately twenty-one days to break old habits and create new ones. Also, I've found that after three weeks of doing these exercises every day my clients start seeing real results and experiencing huge physical breakthroughs that keep them motivated, inspired, and rededicated to making foam rolling a mainstay of their daily routine.

The Roller Workouts

Each day I will guide you through a complete series of warm-ups and foam rolling sequences for both self-massage and sculpting and toning. These movements will alternately decompress the spine and joints (for a taller appearance); smooth out the fascia, elongate and balance the musculature, and build the intrinsic core muscles (for a slimmer appearance); and release stress and smooth out scar tissue (for a younger appearance). Each day includes:

- **Warm-up** exercises to get your body heated and ready to roll.
- **Smooth-out** exercises to release toxins and smooth out fascia and muscle tissue.
- **Reshape** exercises to reconfigure the now-malleable fascia and muscle.
- A listing of **physical benefits** (in the first 10 Series).
- A listing of **emotional benefits** (in the second 10 Series).

- A **Movement Reboot**, which builds on the day's roller series and will help you integrate the benefits of this session into your movement patterns throughout the day (in the first 10 Series).
- A **Self-Care Second**, which demonstrates ways to take care of yourself for enhanced emotional and mental well-being (in the second 10 Series).

Cardio Workouts During the 21-Day Program

I know that you may be hesitant to give up your regular cardio routines over the course of the next twenty-one days. I understand this fear of moving away from the known and concern about caloric intake versus expenditure. But I recommend giving up your cardio routine for at least the first twenty-one days of this program as you drastically improve posture, alignment, body and organ awareness, and muscle movement patterns, while reducing compensation patterns—all of which can be minimized or undone with the wrong kind of cardio work. For example, when you're spinning, your quads are overworking, your legs never go into full extension (which negatively impacts overall alignment), and you're leaned over, which compresses the diaphragm and decreases oxygen intake and carbon dioxide output. All of these factors can hold you back from seeing the maximum results of this program. Not only that, but some types of cardio can ramp up the nervous system and cause a spike in the stress hormone cortisol and in ghrelin, the hormone responsible for increasing appetite. This is counterproductive to what we're trying to do: calm the nervous system, reduce tension, and smooth out thick or overworked areas of the body while also stimulating the lymphatic system, which is responsible for circulating and purifying blood throughout the body, building immunity, releasing toxins, and slimming down.

Of course, the natural concern with cutting cardio is weight gain. I have an answer for that, too. The nervous system is affected when we're overstressed or working really hard, which happens during some cardio workouts. As Jim Karas explains in *The Cardio-Free Diet*, "Cardiovascular workouts do burn a few calories, but far fewer than you think. And the more cardio you do, the hungrier you feel. Not only does cardio fail to help you lose weight, but it kills—it kills your time, your energy, your joints, and your motivation. You burn a few measly calories but then eat twice as many afterward. The result? Weight gain—and lots of it." In other words, the treadmill may say that you just burned 400 calories, but

THE TSY 21-DAY PROGRAM • 11

those calories will be added right back on as soon as you drink that coconut water and latte … *and* you'll still be left feeling hungry. This common scenario is like a Band-Aid—it may cover your wound, but it's not doing anything to actually fix it.

Overextending yourself while working out or doing the wrong type of exercise can actually (and often *does*) make you eat more, not because your body needs more calories but because your nervous system and stress levels are ramped up. We've all heard the phrases "stress eating" and "eating your emotions," right? Avoiding excess cardio allows the body to re-establish its equilibrium and start to remember how much or what types of foods it really needs to feel vibrant and full of vitality, as opposed to going for the quick fix. Mind you, I'm not saying to stop moving altogether. Keep going on walks, taking dance classes, hiking, and swimming. Any activity that feels good and joyful and brings you into your miraculous body is a good thing. When you're aware of your body, you actually know if you're hungry or not—you're more present, more calm and aware, and your appetite naturally and healthily comes into balance and, in some cases, decreases. You start eating for nutrition and a sense of community, rather than to fill a void or compensate for a physical or emotional deficit. You also understand that it's okay to indulge without guilt every once in a while.

I recommend swapping out your existing cardio workout with five to fifteen minutes of rebounding (jumping on a trampoline) after you complete your daily rolling sequences. NASA has done research on rebounding and found that it is 68 percent more effective for cardiovascular health and fat-burning than running.

Plus, it's a fun, effective, low-impact, multidimensional form of cardio exercise wherein the body is working in a three-dimensional way. Not only that, but rebounding is a low-impact way to further stimulate the lymphatic system, decrease stress, build bone density, lift your bum, and bolster immunity, energy levels, and circulation. I have also been told that it even helps release toxic energy if you're sensitive to the vibes of others. Rebounders are relatively inexpensive and can easily be found online and at laurenroxburgh.com. I personally prefer the bellicon brand rebounder. Their quality is second to none, they are silent and solid, they create the lowest impact on the body. If you would prefer not to purchase additional equipment, some other good low-impact cardio options include walking, hiking, swimming, dancing, or any other sort of fluid exercises that allow you to let your body flow naturally.

My clients all lose weight or inches on this program—which befuddles every one of them, not to mention their family and friends. After twenty-one days, I promise you will notice a difference in your body shape and in how your clothes fit. At that point, you can decide if and how much cardio you really want in your workout routine. Think of this next twenty-one days as a way to reset your body and mind for a fresh start.

Day 22 and Beyond

Your journey with foam rolling doesn't have to end on the twenty-second day. Although we'll take twenty-one days to reboot the body, *Taller, Slimmer, Younger* is more than just a three-week program: It is an entrée into a healthier, more fulfilling life. I encourage you to integrate rolling into your everyday life, whether that means continuing to cycle through the 21-day program or using the sequences to complement other fitness activities. You can also use this book as a reference to target specific areas of the body. At the end of this book, you'll find a Glossary of Movements (beginning on page 181), where all of the moves in this program are provided in one place and categorized according to the part of the body they work.

Also be sure to make use of the Roller Rx section (beginning on page 173) and videos available on my website to help alleviate chronic or recurring issues such as anxiety, depression, insomnia, digestion, and more.

Why This Program Works

Now that you have an understanding of *how* the program works, let's talk about *why* it works. In my more than two decades in the fitness and wellness fields, I have studied a wide variety of modalities, including nutrition, yoga, personal training, Structural Integration, and Pilates. It is the latter two that really provide the basis for the foam rolling program you are about to embark on.

Pilates

We tend to think of Pilates as a very modern form of exercise and strength training, but the truth is that it was nearly a century old by the time it became popularized in American culture in the 1980s. It wasn't until then that exercise science and physical therapy finally caught up with the principles of Pilates and what its founder had already known for decades.

Joseph Pilates was born in Germany in 1883. He was a sickly child, and because of his physical weaknesses, Pilates dedicated himself to improving his strength. To accomplish this, he studied a wide range of topics and practices, including everything from yoga, qigong, and Zen Buddhism to ancient Greek and Roman ideals of the human body to the movement of animals. By the age of fourteen, Pilates was so incredibly fit, so balanced and toned, that he served as a model for anatomy charts! He came to realize from his studies and self-experimentation that the "modern" lifestyle of bad posture and inefficient breathing is at the base of poor health. And this was before the turn of the nineteenth century!

While placed under forced internment in England during World War I, Pilates began to teach soldiers the exercises he had developed, in the process unwittingly devising the universal system of floor exercises known today as matwork. A few years later, Pilates was transferred to another military camp, where he became a caretaker and healer for the many wounded and sick soldiers. To rehabilitate them, Pilates devised transformative equipment crafted of springs from hospital beds to support and encourage movement and to rebuild balanced muscle tone. Pilates equipment today is not much different than it was when Pilates developed it for those first practitioners. His equipment simultaneously challenges and supports the body while the body learns to move more efficiently. Perhaps you see where I'm going with this: The foam roller does the same thing!

Structural Integration

Rolfing, Structural Integration, and Hellerwork are all forms of alignment and fascia-based bodywork that originated from another pioneer, Ida Pauline Rolf. She was basically a female rocket scientist who studied how the human body related to gravity. Rolf was born in New York City in 1896 and, like Pilates, experienced childhood health issues that set her along a path to find answers.

Rolf dedicated her life to studying and experimenting with different systems of healing and manipulation, exploring many forms of alternative healing in the process, including homeopathy, hatha yoga, movement techniques, osteopathy, and chiropractic work. She came to realize that all of these healing modalities are rooted in proper alignment, increasing one's life force, and improving the balance and efficiency of one's anatomical structure. She fused these ideas together to create Structural Integration, which is a "holistic system of soft tissue manipulation and movement education that organize[s] the whole body in gravity." Her foundation in science and medical research allowed her to ensure this unique approach could be scientifically validated.

Structural Integration revolves around a 10 Series program, which is typically done in a progression of ten sessions (sometimes referred to as the recipe), with each session addressing different parts of the body. The ultimate purpose of this system is to educate the body to have better alignment and function within gravity. Rolf came up with the theory that bound-up fascia (or connective tissue; more on this below) often restrict opposing muscles from functioning in a balanced way. Through bodywork, she aimed to manually separate bound-up fascia in order to lengthen, elongate, and align, thus allowing for graceful and effective movement. What I love about her research is that while she was developing her approach, Rolf found a connection between emotions and the soft tissues of the body. This led her to the idea that chronic patterns of muscular tension can store negative emotions and stress, which perpetuate the influence of those emotions in an individual's body and even in his or her personality.

As a Structural Integration practitioner myself, I base my program on this ten-session recipe philosophy, with one significant tweak. In Structural Integration, a practitioner performs bodywork on a patient. In my program, the practitioner is empowered to use the foam roller him- or herself and learn how to self-heal, align, strenghten, and prevent injury, tension, and pain every single day.

Fascia

In retrospect, it's a little bit mind-boggling how ahead of her time Ida Rolf actually was. Despite the fact that she had theorized about and was working with fascia in the early twentieth century, it wasn't until 2007 that the medical and scientific communities came to understand the importance of fascia. Prior to that point, fascia was considered nothing more than a nuisance because it encased muscle and thus had to be removed in order for scientists and medical students to examine muscle composition and function. That's right: Until just a few years ago, medical schools were *literally* disregarding fascia during cadaver dissections because it was simply considered waste material. In terms of fitness, it turns out that this knowledge and understanding of fascia is as revolutionary as discovering that the world is round instead of flat—it changes *everything.* The science and medical worlds suddenly understood that, far from being disposable, fascia is actually nothing short of critical because it helps to create the shape of our bodies. Not only that, but fascia is the largest and richest sensory organ in the human body, which makes it essential for maintaining alignment, vitality, and function.

So, what is fascia? Basically, it's like a very thin wetsuit just under the skin that wraps around the entire body and also around each individual muscle. It keeps everything in place and connected like a matrix, including our organs, muscles, tendons, ligaments, attachments to joints, and of course, our posture. It connects and separates things in the body.

By nature, fascia is malleable (although, in an unhealthy state, it becomes stagnant, rigid, and knotted up, and lacks a healthy, oxygenated blood supply). Imagine a sponge and how springy, stretchy, and resilient it is when it's wet versus how hard, stiff, and dense it is without moisture. Juicy, thin, hydrated, and lubricated fascia (think Saran Wrap) is happy fascia … and that makes for a happier and lighter person. For better or for worse, fascia changes form based on our actions, movements, and patterns. If we repeat a certain motion over and over again, our fascia will begin to adjust its shape in a way that reflects that movement or movement pattern—think about "text neck" and how it can lead to a hunchback. Because the fascia is an interconnected web of tissue that covers the entire body, when one area of the body is misshapen or out of alignment, it naturally affects other connected areas of the body, throwing them out of alignment, too. Healthy fascia is thin, smooth, hydrated, and resilient, like plastic wrap; unhealthy fascia is thick and holds toxins and stress. It's this unhealthy fascia that we think of as scar tissue, thickness, and knots.

It follows that fascia is integral in our efforts to achieve both long, lean muscle and proper alignment. It's no coincidence that these are two of the most critical components in creating a taller, slimmer, younger physique. So how do we manipulate this malleable fascia into its healthiest, most optimal form?

Along with increased body awareness and posture, there is one simple tool that allows us to reach these goals. You've probably guessed by now that I'm talking about the fantastic foam roller.

How the Foam Roller Works

The roller is the best tool that allows you to independently remove the stored-up density and toxins in the tissues—and specifically, the fascia—while simultaneously hydrating the tissue with oxygenated blood and fluid. The end result is healthy, malleable tissue just waiting to be worked into tip-top shape. The roller delves into the fascia in much the same way bodywork does, flushing the toxins from the fascia; smoothing the thick, dense scar tissue; and hydrating the connective tissue to create a smoother, healthier, leaner, and more vibrant appearance. All of this also helps reformulate the structure of the muscles into a sculpted, sleeker, leaner, more malleable form. Once you're working with this healthy, shapeable tissue, you can then use the combination of lengthening, toning moves, and the rolling fascia to create long, sinewy muscle—in other words, *healthy and balanced* muscle—and fascia that ultimately give your body a beautiful longer, leaner, more youthful shape.

The roller helps you use and sculpt your intrinsic core and postural muscles … or, once again, those graceful ballerina muscles. When incorporated with the lengthening and toning Pilates moves, the foam roller encourages your body to access the stabilizing or age-delaying muscles. In order to balance your body while using the roller, you must "turn on" your core and intrinsic muscles. Generally speaking, these muscles are extremely difficult to connect with; however, when balance is brought into the mix, you turn them on naturally to stabilize yourself. These are the muscles that will keep you slim, strong, and fit, so activating and using them is essential to sculpting the healthy and sexy body you crave. The foam roller essentially offers an on-switch that makes this connection simple.

• • •

I'm confident that you, just as my clients have been, will be blown away by how much your entire body and life both shift in the course of three weeks. Not only will you rediscover a taller, slimmer, younger physique, but you will also discover how mind and body work in tandem. It has been said that our physical bodies are a direct reflection of our emotional selves. These sequences will demonstrate how mindful movement and proer breath can enhance not only our physical state but also our emotional well-being.

Now … let's get rolling!

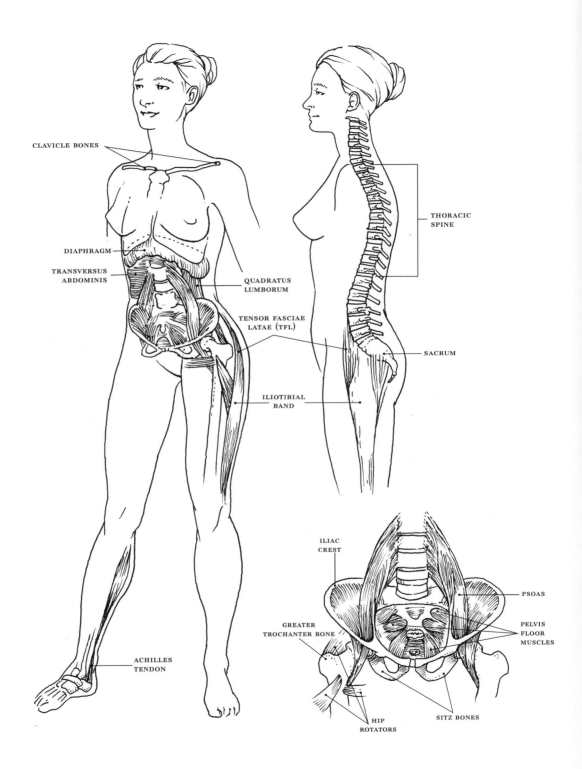

CLAVICLE BONES

DIAPHRAGM

TRANSVERSUS
ABDOMINIS

QUADRATUS
LUMBORUM

TENSOR FASCIAE
LATAE (TFL)

ILIOTIBIAL
BAND

ACHILLES
TENDON

THORACIC
SPINE

SACRUM

ILIAC
CREST

PSOAS

PELVIS
FLOOR
MUSCLES

GREATER
TROCHANTER BONE

SITZ BONES

HIP
ROTATORS

Aligned Body

DAYS 1–10

10 SERIES WITH A PHYSICAL FOCUS

For the first ten days of this program, we'll focus on the more physical aspects of our well-being. We'll discuss alignment, core connection, and a more balanced musculature. As I always tell my clients, this program is definitely about aesthetic benefits, but it goes far deeper than that. With this work, we're digging deep to change the biomechanics of your body in ways that will reduce pain, stress, and tension while simultaneously elongating, leaning you out, and helping you stand taller. Through this integrative method, we can literally melt the years and inches away and increase your height anywhere from a half to one and a half inches. Once you have achieved this height you will immediately look ten pounds slimmer. The work you're about to learn will help your body function more efficiently *all* of the time—of course when you're actually working out, but also when you're sitting at your desk or in traffic, walking from Point A to Point B, putting groceries away, and even sleeping.

Ten days from now, your body will look and feel better and be well on its way to humming like a well-oiled machine!

A Word About the Way You Stand

In many of my exercise instructions I ask you to stand with your feet "hip width apart." In the photos that accompany my instructions, you may think that my feet look placed more narrowly than what you might traditionally think as "hip width" but anatomically speaking, it means I want you to align your feet with your sitz bones or hip joints. In other words, follow my lead—I really do mean *only* hip width, and that is going to look and feel slightly more narrow than you might have guessed.

Roller Pro Tip

Finding Your Neutral Spine

Lie back on your mat with your knees bent and heels hip width apart. See those three bony landmarks created by your hip bones and pubic bone? When your spine is neutral, you could easily balance a level across all three of them. This is a neutral spine, and it's the form you want not only while you're exercising but also while you walk, sit, and stand. Once you identify your neutral spine, you've mastered one of the great secrets of accessing your core more efficiently and effectively!

We may talk about straightening the spine a lot, but the reality is that everyone has a few healthy curves, and some of us naturally have more of a curve than others, based on how our body is built. Humans don't actually have straight spines. In order to help the body deal with different gravitational stresses, we actually have three curves (the cervical, thoracic, and lumbar), which allow the spine to support more weight than a straight spine would. These healthy curves also help prevent compression or squishing of the spine..

DAY 1

Breath of Life

Chest, Shoulders, and Arms

We'll start this program at the very beginning: learning how to breathe. This is essential for physical, mental, and emotional health.

Hunched, slumped, and poor posture are all often directly linked to incorrect breathing. Fully expanding and filling the lungs encourages the spine to lengthen. Try taking a deep breath and see how you naturally sit or stand taller. Awesome, right? And here's an incredible statistic: Our bodies are designed to release 70 percent of their toxins through breath (better than a juice cleanser). I know it sounds almost *too* easy, but this simple tweak can actually help regulate weight, flush toxins, improve digestion, promote better sleep, and create a taller stature!

When you are breathing correctly, not only do you exercise more efficiently, but you also *live* more efficiently. The roller exercises today will focus on the rib cage, collarbone, chest, neck, shoulders, diaphragm, and lungs. All of this will help build a heightened awareness of your breath. It also brings awareness to your posture and any tension or blockages in the body, and expands the chest for deeper breath, decreased stress, and a calmer nervous system. By breathing more efficiently and increasing the oxygen intake, your body releases more CO_2, which helps burn excess fat and regulates all of your systems. The more fat you burn, the more you slim down.

I promised results, and I plan to deliver. On day 1, we're starting off with a movement that will immediately set you on the road to feeling taller, slimmer, and younger!

Standing Chest Expansion

• Come to a standing position with your feet hip width apart and soft knees. Hold your arms out to the side with a slight bend in the elbows, palms facing forward and fingers pointing up.
• Inhale as you reach your right arm behind you and twist your body to the right to expand your chest, lungs, and arms.
• Exhale as you come back through the center and reach your left arm behind you as you twist to the left.

Repeat this movement ten times.

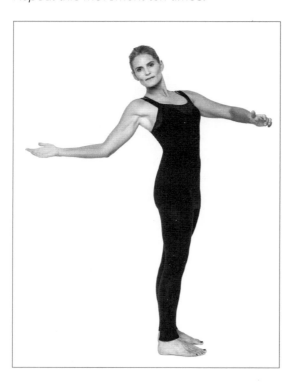
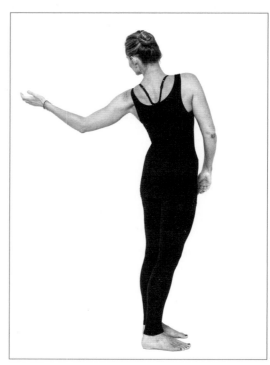

SMOOTH-OUT

Snow Angels

- Lie on the roller with your spine supported from head to tailbone. Begin with your arms extended down by your sides, with the palms of your hands facing up to open and expand the chest.
- Inhale deeply as you reach your arms up overhead slowly and with control, keeping them as close to the mat as possible and parallel to the floor.
- Exhale completely as you draw your arms back down to your sides.

Repeat this movement eight times.

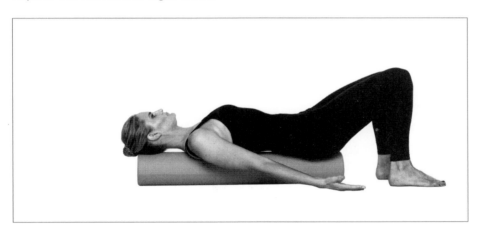

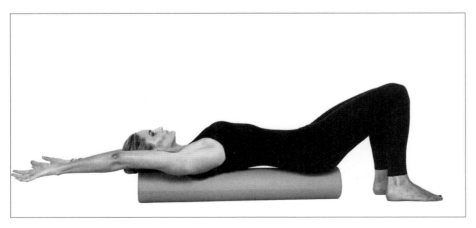

Diaphragm Release

- Place the roller underneath the bottom of your shoulder blades (at the bra line, for the ladies). Gently interlace your fingers and bring your hands behind your head to support your neck. Place your feet on the floor, with knees bent and feet hip width apart.
- Inhale as you arch your thoracic spine (or middle to upper back) over the roller.
- Exhale as you curl back up as if you were doing a crunch, squeezing all the air out of your stomach.

Repeat this movement eight to ten times.

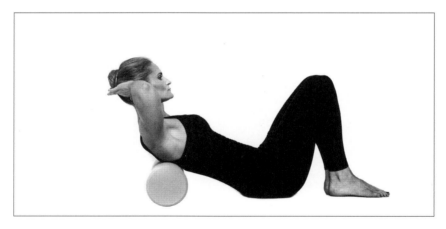

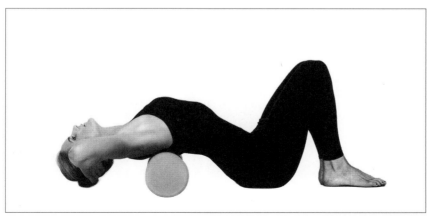

RESHAPE

Reverse Push-Through

- Place the roller horizontally about a foot behind you. Sit up tall with your legs long out in front of you. Reach behind you to place your palms facedown on the roller, thumbs pointing out.

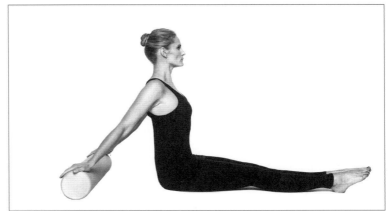

- Inhale as you scoop your tail under, placing some weight onto the roller. As you roll back, scoop your belly as the roller rolls up your wrists and forearms to just below your elbow joints. You will end up with a long spine and your arms, shoulders, and chest stretched open.

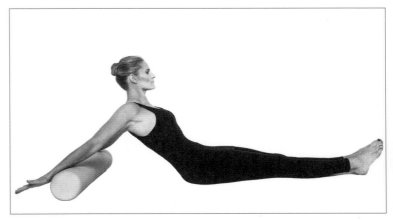

- Exhale as you slowly roll back up to a tall spine, sitting on your sitz bones.

Repeat this movement six times.

BREATH OF LIFE • 25

Rolling Swan

- Lie belly-down on the mat, with arms long in front of you and the roller placed just below your elbow joints, thumbs facing up. Reach your heels away from your heart to feel oppositional energy and decompress your spine.
- Inhale and roll the roller toward you, extending your spine and lifting your heart as you roll your shoulders back (taking care to keep your glutes relaxed the entire time so you don't jam your lower back while lifting up). Be sure to pull your abs up and in to support your back and elongate the front of your body.
- Exhale as you slowly resist on the way down, returning to the position you started in.

Repeat this movement eight times.

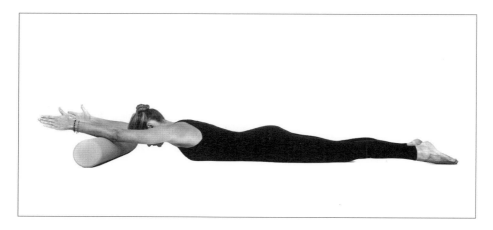

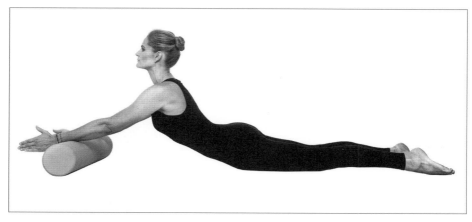

Physical Benefits

- Reduces tension in shoulders.
- Calms the nervous system.
- Increases oxygen intake, which boosts metabolism and regulates hormones.
- Creates a younger, more relaxed appearance.
- Helps you stand taller.

MOVEMENT REBOOT

With just a few minutes' practice per day, you can dramatically increase your lung capacity, improve your posture, and reduce stress by doing what I call *umbrella breathing*. To do this, visualize your lungs as a three-dimensional umbrella. Imagine you are opening the umbrella by taking a full inhale, during which you expand your lungs to the greatest degree possible, expanding the front, back, and sides of the ribs. Pause at the top of your breath, then slowly release a full, calm exhale (as if you were sighing in relief). Pause again at the bottom of your breath and repeat five to ten times.

Getting Grounded

Feet, Ankles, and Lower Legs

hink about a healthy tree and how its strong, firm roots allow its trunk to stand tall and its branches to dance in the breeze. Today we're going to find proper alignment in the lower body, which serves as our connection to teh earth, creating the solid foundation we need to stand taller and bring more fluidity into the upper body. To do this, we'll focus on the feet and legs, balancing our body weight through the feet by aligning them with our knees and ankles. This sequence will ultimately help you stand more upright while also feeling more grounded, not only resulting in a taller appearance but also allowing you to engage your core for a slimmer physique. Double win!

WARM-UP

Heel Lifts

- Stand with your feet hip width apart and arms raised overhead.
- As you inhale, pull your belly in and up as you slowly lift your heels off the floor, keeping your ankles stable.
- Exhale as you slowly lower your heels back down to the floor.

Repeat this movement eight times.

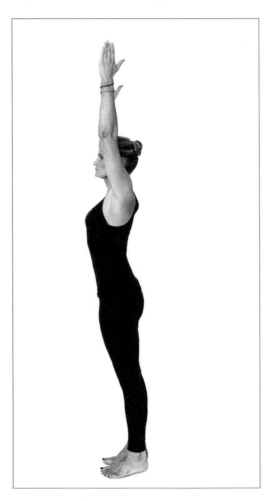
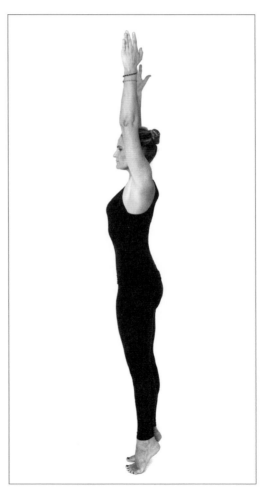

SMOOTH-OUT

Foot Roll

- Place the ball of your left foot on the roller six inches in front of your standing foot while balancing on your right foot.
- Inhale as you press your foot into the roller, moving the roller from your arch to the front of your heel. Apply as much pressure as you can, to the point where you feel that hurts-so-good sensation.
- Exhale and roll back to your starting position.

Repeat three sets of eight rolls on each side. The roller should be placed under the center of the arch of your foot.

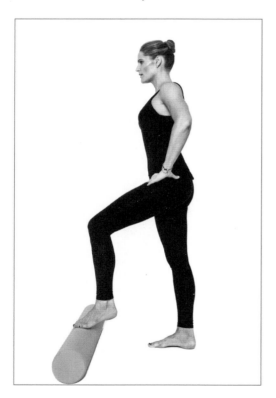
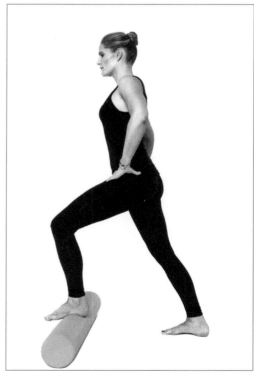

Kneeling Lunge Shin Roll

- Come to a kneeling lunge on your mat, beginning with your right leg forward and bent at a 90-degree angle. Place the roller just below the kneecap of your left leg. Place your hands slightly in front of your shoulders on either side of your foot.

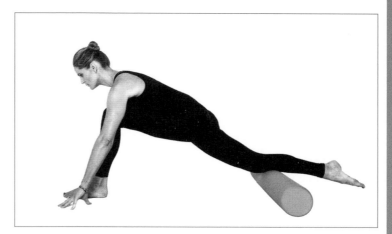

- Inhale as you ground through your front foot and pull yourself forward, straightening your back leg as the roller rolls down your shin. (Note: exhale as your return to the starting position)

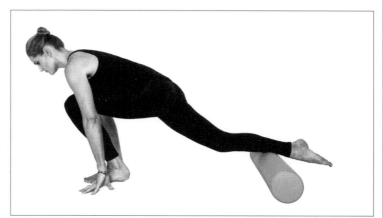

Repeat this movement eight to ten times per leg.

Roller Rx

High Heel Relief

This movement stretches the hips and releases any blockages in the acupressure points along the shin. This in turn releases tension in the lower legs and feet.

Standing Footwork

- Stand with your feet turned out. Stand the roller up in front of you and place both of your hands on top of the roller for a little bit of support.
- Lift your heels so that you're standing on your toes. Keep weight even through all five toes of each foot (don't collapse inward or outward).
- Keeping your heels lifted, ankles stable, and spine neutral, inhale as you bend your knees wide and lower down a few inches.
- Continue to keep your heels lifted as you exhale and straighten your knees (without locking them), returning to the starting position.

Repeat this movement eight times.

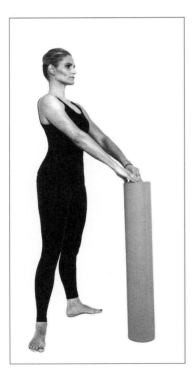 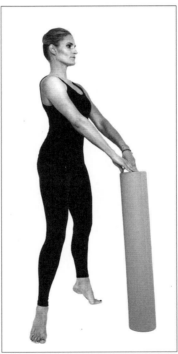 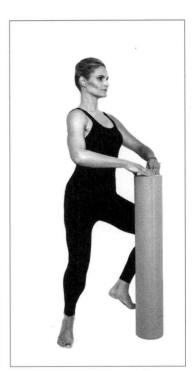

Core Stability Footwork

- Lie on the roller with a neutral spine, with the roller supporting you from head to tailbone. Place your forearms on either side of the roller to stabilize. Lift your legs with your knees bent at a 90-degree angle, heels together, toes apart.
- Lift your shoulder blades off the roller and curl up over your bra line, keeping a long neck.
- Maintaining your curl, inhale as you slowly extend your legs out to a 45-degree angle, maintaining a neutral spine.
- Exhale as you slowly draw your legs back in to return to the starting position.

Repeat this movement eight to ten times.

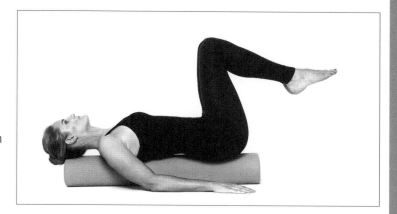

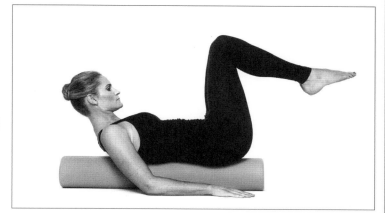

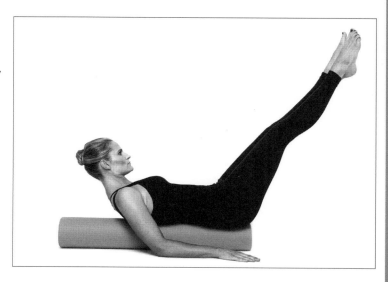

Physical Benefits

- Fosters connection to the feet, which helps connect to the core.
- Strengthens feet.
- Increases stability and balance.
- Creates a suspension system in the body.
- Takes pressure off the knees, hips, and lower back.
- Speeds up reaction time.
- Improves your ability to jump.
- Reduces varicose veins.

MOVEMENT REBOOT

We can find that truly grounded and stable connection to the entire foot by thinking of its three primary grounding points, which I call the *tripod foot*. Come to a standing position and feel yourself grounding down in those areas right underneath your pinkie toe, your big toe, and across the bottom of your heel. Some people have a tendency to lean forward, which can result in a feeling of not living in the present moment and perpetually being on to the next thing. Others may collapse inward or ride the outside of their feet, which can cause imbalances throughout the entire body.

Keeping these three grounding points in mind, begin to walk. Make sure that you're using your *entire* foot, setting your heel down, then rolling over the arch, and ending the step at the root of your toes. Not only will this properly engage your muscles and keep you in alignment, but it's also a good reminder to remain in the moment. Rather than letting your brain wander off to your to-do list, your destination, or anywhere else that isn't right here and now, use the awareness of your movement to remain in the present moment.

DAY 3

Long and Strong Legs

Legs

Get ready to break out those skinny jeans that have been gathering dust in the back of your closet. Today you'll work on flushing toxins, narrowing and leaning out the legs and thighs, and elongating the entire leg from top to bottom for that long, lean skinny-jeans look. You'll reduce the bulkiness in the thighs and calves that is caused by overdeveloped or thick quadriceps (this should sound familiar to you high-impact cardio nuts out there!). You'll create balanced and uniform 3-D development of the leg muscles, hitting the front, back, and sides. *And* you'll reduce the appearance of cellulite and saddlebags by activating and strengthening both legs equally. Are you excited? Because you should be!

Chair Pose

- Come to a standing position with your feet hip width apart. Reach your arms up to the ceiling with palms facing in toward each other.
- Inhale as you bend your knees as if you're going to sit down in a chair. Keeping your weight equally balanced between both feet, activate your entire foot by spreading your toes and pressing into your pinkie toes, big toes, and heels. Stay in this position for twenty seconds, inhaling and exhaling deeply while holding this pose.

Repeat this movement five times.

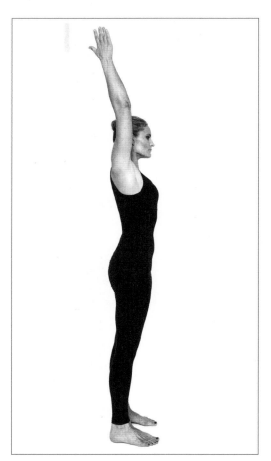
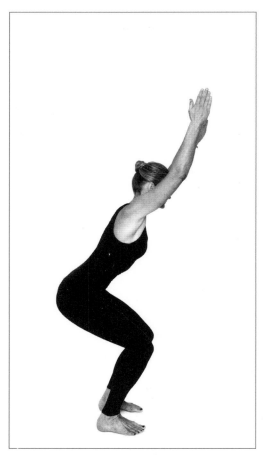

SMOOTH-OUT

Calf Roll

- Sit on your mat with your legs close together and the roller placed under both of your calves, right below the knee joint. Place your hands palms-down on the floor a few inches out from either side of your hips, fingers pointing outward. Press down into your hands to lift your bottom off the mat, keeping your calves balanced on the roller. Make sure to draw your shoulders down and back to avoid hunching.

- Continue pressing your hands down and engage your core, exhaling to slowly drive your body weight forward so that the roller stops right above the ankle.

- As you inhale, slowly draw the roller back so that it stops right below the knee.

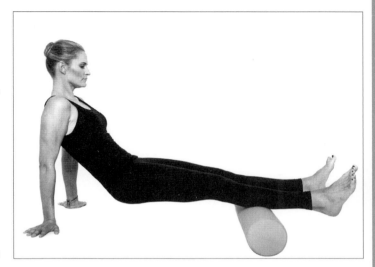

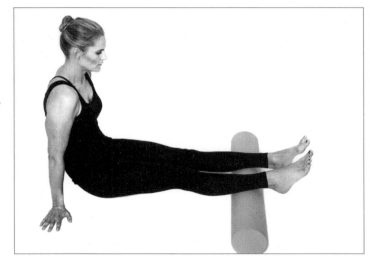

Repeat three sets of eight rolls. The roller should be placed under the center of your calves for the first set, the inner edge of the calves for the second set, and the outer edge of the calves for the third set.

Back of Thigh Roll

- Sit on your mat with the roller under your hamstrings, right above the knee joint. Place your hands on the mat behind you, with fingertips slightly turned out. Press your hands into the mat to lift your bottom off the floor, and engage your core.
- Keep your shoulders back and inhale as you roll the roller up the back of your thighs.
- Exhale as you roll back down to the starting position.

Repeat this movement eight to ten times.

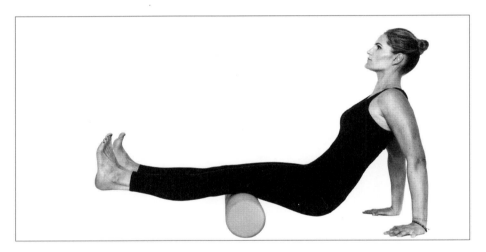

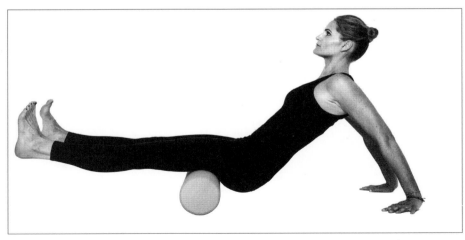

Front of Thigh Roll

- Place the roller above the knees. Bring your elbows to the mat about two inches behind your shoulders and make fists. Engage your core to prop yourself up and protect your lower back.
- Using your arms and core, exhale as you pull yourself forward as the roller rolls up the front of your thighs.
- Inhale as you press the roller down to just above the front of your knees.

Repeat this movement eight to ten times.

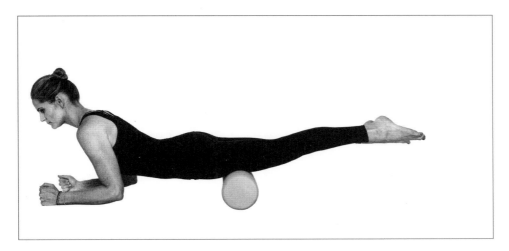

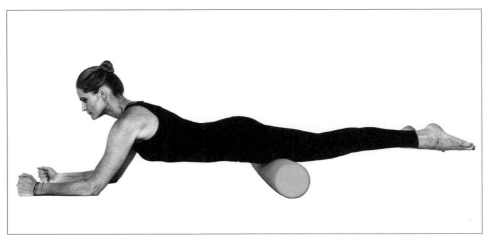

Thigh Stretch

- Kneel on the mat with your knees hip width apart, big toes together. Bring the roller over your head, placing a hand on either side of it. Keep your shoulders down and chest open. Establish a neutral spine (see the box on page 20) and maintain a stable spine and pelvis throughout this exercise.
- As you inhale, begin hinging back from your knee joints. Engage your inner thighs and pull your belly in and up to keep the weight off your knees. Hold the pose for three seconds.
- Exhale as you press your shins down and slowly float back up to your starting position.

Repeat this movement eight to ten times.

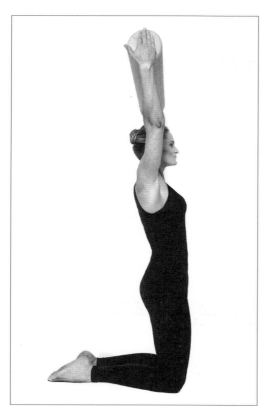
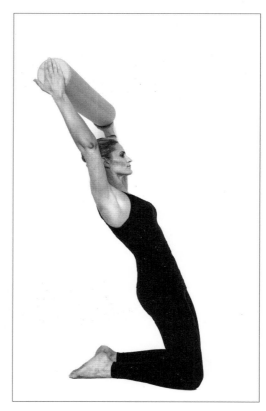

Stomach Massage

- Sit up tall on the mat with your knees bent, heels together and toes apart. Place your toes on the roller and engage your core, thighs, and arms. Reach your arms out to a 45-degree angle, keeping your shoulder blades drawn down toward your hips. (In other words, don't hunch your neck—it should feel nice and long, not scrunched up.)
- Engage your arm muscles and inhale as you extend your legs long, pressing the roller away from you and simultaneously rolling your spine into a C-shape while pulling your belly in and up.
- As you exhale, engage your core and draw the roller back in to the point where your knees are bent and your spine is tall.

Repeat this exercise eight to ten times.

Physical Benefits

- Aligns the legs and hip bones.
- Elongates thigh muscles.
- Reduces bulkiness in the thighs and calves.
- Increases circulation.
- Leans out the legs.
- Reduces cellulite.
- Reduces saddlebags.

MOVEMENT REBOOT

Think back to the beginning of this chapter when you realigned your feet so that your toes were pointing forward, rather than in or out. This will build the muscles of your legs into a longer, leaner shape, as well as making them more balanced and toned. As you move throughout your day, try to remember to look down every now and then, making a concerted effort to place your feet as close to parallel as possible, toes pointing forward to balance out the musculature of your legs when you stand and walk. If you remind yourself often enough, soon this will become habit … and your muscles will show it! Especially be aware of how you drive with your right goot on the gas …

Waist-Shrinking Bikini Session

Waist, Lower Back, and Sides

This sequence is all about creating length, balance, and a sense of three dimensions in the sides of the body. To get there, we'll focus on the fascia and muscle tone all the way from the knee up to the ear. Thanks to our old friend gravity, many of us experience an all-too-typical pattern of ribs collapsing onto the hips. This results in an unhealthy and uncomfortable posture, squishes the organs, and makes the waistline wider. All of this affects the area of your body that is involved in respiration, digestion, elimination, and reproduction. You can probably see how it's nothing short of essential to release any existing compression in the side and waist areas for true vitality. There are some other fringe benefits, too. In this session you'll reveal your hourglass waist, shrink your waist, and align your sides by releasing tension in your shoulders, arms, and side body. Taller, slimmer, and more vital, here you come!

Standing Side Bends

- Stand up tall with your feet hip width apart and knees soft. With arms shoulder-width apart, hold the roller overhead.
- Inhale to reach up and over to the right to open up the left side of your body.
- Exhale to reach up and over to the left to open up the right side of your body.

Repeat this movement five times on each side, alternating sides.

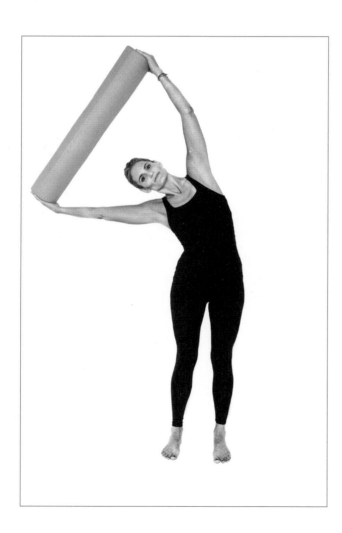

Figure Four

- Sit on the roller and reach your right arm behind you with your right hand on the mat, thumb out to the side. Cross your right ankle over your left knee to form a figure four. Press your left hand down into your right inner thigh.

- Shift your weight slightly over to the left hip/glute area and roll back and forth a few inches in each direction.

- Next, roll in circles to help increase circulation and blood flow and to reduce congestion.

Repeat this movement on the other side.

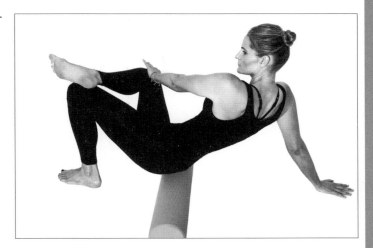

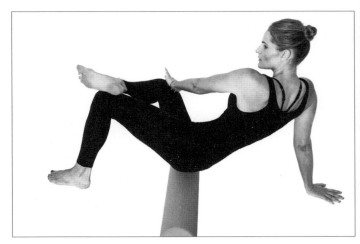

12th-Rib Roll

- Bring your left hip down to the mat and place the roller at your waistline (below your left lower ribs and above your left hip). Stack your left elbow under your left shoulder and bring your left forearm to the mat so it's running parallel to the roller. Keep your left hip on the mat, bend your right knee, and ground your right foot in front of your left knee.

- Inhale as you gently rock forward, leaning and twisting your upper body toward the roller.

- Exhale as you roll your ribs back to center.

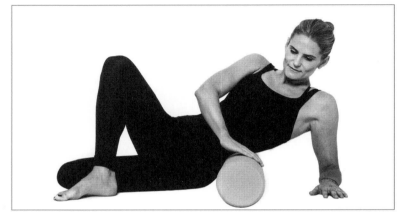

Repeat this movement six times on each side, alternating sides.

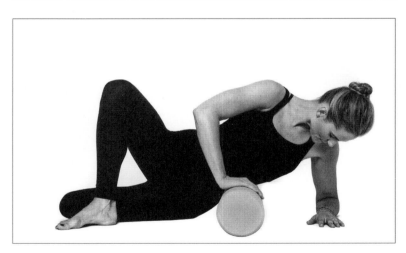

RESHAPE

Hourglass

- Place the roller under your left leg, just above the left anklebone, and cross your right leg over your left. Place your left elbow directly under your left shoulder, with your forearm flat on the floor and fingers spread; reach your right arm up and slightly back. Press down into your left leg and forearm, using this traction to lift your side body (or "hourglass") off the floor, taking care to keep the roller stable as you lift.
- Inhaling, resist as you lower your hips and right arm down, hovering a few inches above the mat.
- Exhale as you lift with your waist to return to your starting position.

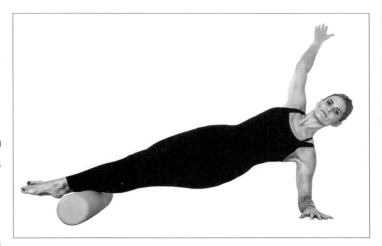

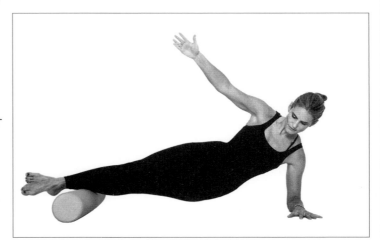

Repeat this exercise eight to ten times before switching to the other side.

Side Kicks

• Hinge your legs at a 45-degree angle, with your heels together. Place the roller between your right lower rib cage and right hip. Bend your left elbow to bring your left hand lightly behind your head; bring your right forearm to the mat with your thumb pointing up, and your right elbow slightly behind your right shoulder.
• Inhale as you use your belly to lift your legs, maintaining your upper body posture.
• Exhale as you lower your legs, leaving them to hover slightly over the mat.

Repeat this motion ten times on each side.

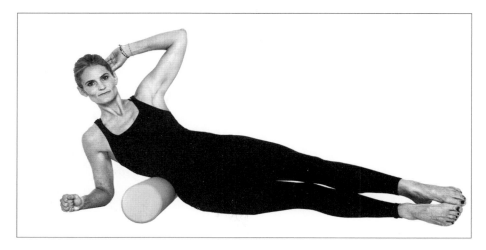

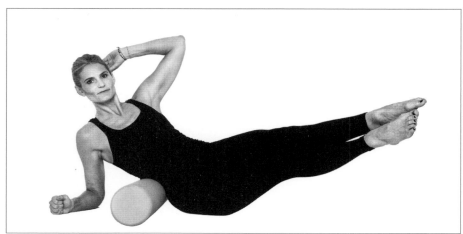

Physical Benefits

- Reshapes the sides of the body.
- Reduces tension in the lower back.
- Reveal hourglass waist.
- Shrinks and elongates the waist.
- Aligns the sides by releasing tension in the entire trunk and sides of the body.
- Promotes digestion and elimination.

MOVEMENT REBOOT

Considering we walk an average of 5,000 to 10,000 steps per day, what better practice *is* there than walking to whittle your waist, tone your core, and wring out your organs? Find new fluidity and a sense of ease as you walk by allowing your ribs to rotate in opposition to your hips (called transverse motion—or as *I* call it, "channeling your inner supermodel"). Walking in this manner will continue the work of establishing length in your side body and creating freedom for your ribs to gracefully rotate away from your hips. You're simultaneously working the core, standing taller, and looking younger with this simple movement modification.

Strong, Smiling Booty

Glutes

The booty muscles are so important in keeping us healthy, strong, and efficient that I actually consider them part of the core. As most of you ladies are probably well aware, the tush is an area where women tend to store fat. While fat storage here is normal and healthy, too much fat on top of the largest muscle in the body (the gluteus maximus) can result in a more saggy tush. Plus, this area can become droopy, flat, and start frowning with age, a look most of us would like to avoid. Let's defy gravity and keep that tush high and smiling!

If you're like me, you're probably tired of performing endless squats and lunges in hopes of slimming and shaping your derriere. Well, this session will help reveal the balanced tush you've always wanted minus the squats and lunges, while simultaneously providing your body with more stability and less compression of your joints.

Bridge

- Lie on your back, bend your knees, and place the roller under the balls of your feet, feet parallel. Reach your arms long by your sides.
- Keeping the roller stable, inhale as you start to roll up your spine one vertebra at a time while scooping your belly.
- Exhale up to a neutral spine bridge position.
- Slowly lower yourself back down to the starting position, taking a full round of breath to get there.

Repeat this movement eight times.

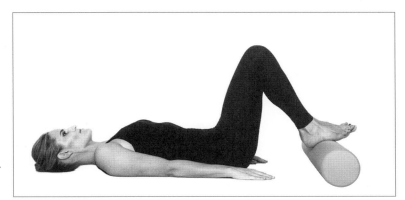

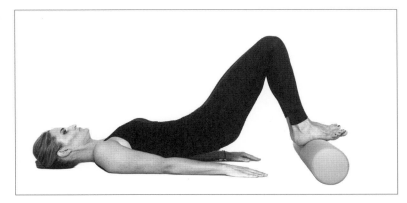

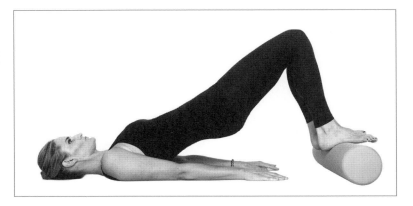

Inverted Tush Roll

- Slide the roller under your hips/sacrum (the triangular bone at the base of your spine), just above the tailbone. Lift your knees up so they are hovering directly over your hips. Hold either side of the roller.
- Inhale as you twist and draw your knees over to the left at a 45-degree angle.
- Exhale, using your core to return to center.

Repeat this movement eight times on each side, alternating sides.

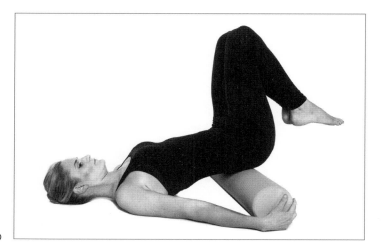

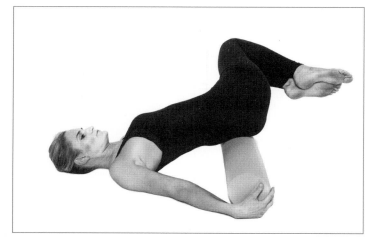

Inverted Figure Four Circles

- Lie down on the mat and come to a bridge position, sliding the roller under your hips/sacrum. Hold either end of the roller to stabilize yourself. Bend and lift your knees, and then cross your right ankle over your left knee, creating an inverted figure four.
- Inhale as you roll to the right while keeping your ribs and shoulders stable.
- Exhale as you circle down and back around up to the starting position.

Repeat this motion five times on each side, alternating sides.

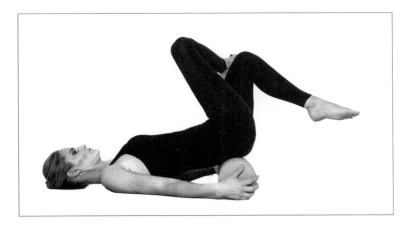

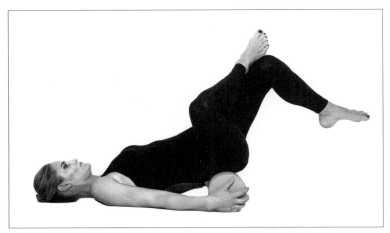

Grasshopper

- Place your lower thighs (right above your kneecaps) on the roller and your hands directly under your shoulders, fingers pointing forward. Inhale to bring your spine into extension, looking straight ahead.
- Exhale and bend your elbows to lower down, hovering over the mat.
- Inhale to return to your starting position.

Repeat this movement eight to ten times.

Roller Pro Tip

As you inhale and lift in this pose, be sure to engage your hamstrings to keep pressure out of your lower back. Think of your body as a teeter-totter: You want to keep your weight equal as you go up and down.

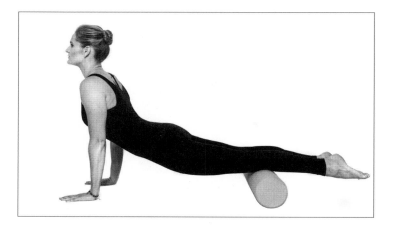

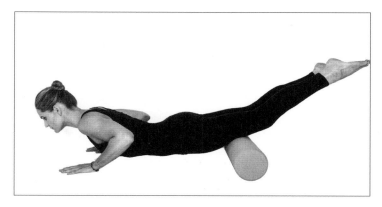

High Frog

- Press the soles of your feet together so that your knees are bent out to the sides, and place the sides of your ankles on the roller.
- Inhale and press your pubic bone up to the ceiling, engaging your core and keeping the roller stable.
- Exhale as you lower and hover your hips over the mat.

Repeat this movement five to eight times.

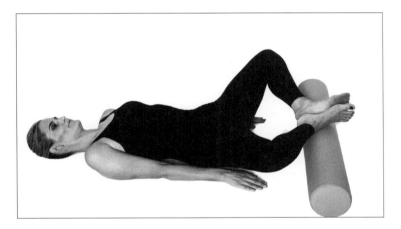

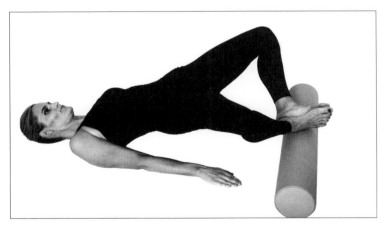

MOVEMENT REBOOT

As a culture, we are a bunch of tight-asses—literally. When we get stressed or tense, we tend to clench our butt ... and most of us are stressed or tense way too often. Butt-gripping is actually one of the reasons that our tush starts to sag with age; it gets stuck in a tucked-under position. This is exacerbated by the fact that we do a lot more sitting than we are designed for these days. Check in with your booty right now: Do you feel yourself gripping? When the butt does its gripping thing, all the tissue around the area where you're holding tension will thicken, tighten, compress, sag, and sometimes even cause pain. Not only that, but over-use of these muscles can shut down healing movement throughout the entire spine. Make a point of checking in with your tush throughout the day (especially during moments of tension or stress), and relaxing its muscles whenever you can so that you learn to use the muscles when you need them and let them chill when you don't.

DAY 6

Release and Love the Hips

Hips

Our hips are lovely, curvy, and sexy. But they're also susceptible to blockages, tightness, rigidity (both physically and emotionally), and even cellulite, which doesn't feel so sexy. Opening, lengthening, and releasing soft tissue tension toxins from your hips will help free your entire body from pain, compression, and heaviness. Not only that, but elongating and strengthening your hips creates more flexibility, more balanced tone, and a greater fluidity of movement. It even improves spine and leg circulation and alignment.

Low Lunge with Thigh Extension

- Come to the mat in a bent knee lunge, beginning with your right foot forward, knee stacked directly over your ankle at a 90-degree angle. Place your left leg behind you with the top of your foot flat on the mat. Slowly lift your core and left arm up, keeping your shoul-ders relaxed as you twist your body to the right and reach around to the back of your left thigh to feel the front of your hip and psoas stretch and lengthen while you breathe into it.

- Gently deepen into the stretch for about thirty seconds as you continue to breathe slowly and steadily. This movement will allow you to go deeper and send oxygenated blood to the hips.

Repeat this movement on the other side.

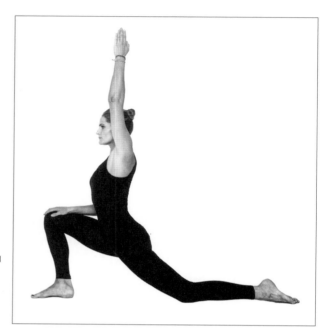

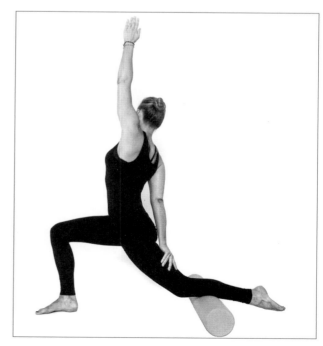

SMOOTH-OUT

Side of Hip Roll

- Sit down with one hip placed on the mat. Prop yourself up by grounding your lower hand on the mat with your wrist crease directly under your shoulder. Place the roller under your seated hip, edging it toward your outer hip. Bend your top leg to ground your foot down in front of the extended leg for support and leverage.
- Use your grounded hand and upper leg to move the roller a few inches up and down the outer hip and thigh, stopping just above the knee. Exhale deeply as you draw in and inhale as you extend.

Repeat this movement on each side eight to ten times.

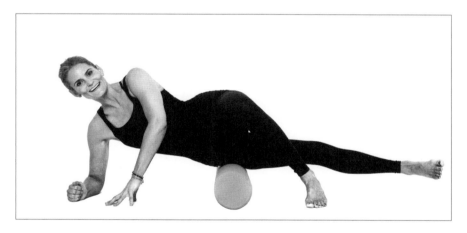

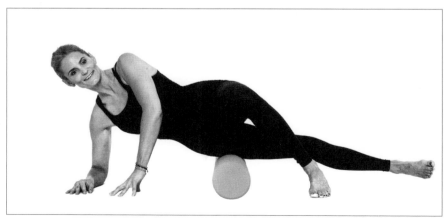

Figure Four

- Sit on the roller and reach your right arm behind you with your right hand on the mat, thumb out to the side. Cross your right ankle over your left knee in a figure four position. Press your left hand down into your right inner thigh.
- Shift your weight slightly over to the left hip/glute area and roll back and forth a few inches in each direction.
- Next roll in circles to help increase circulation and blood flow and to reduce congestion.

Repeat this movement on the other side.

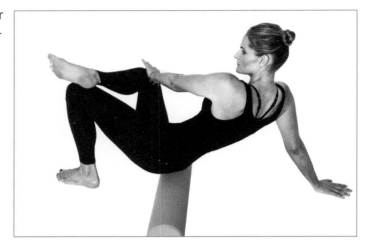

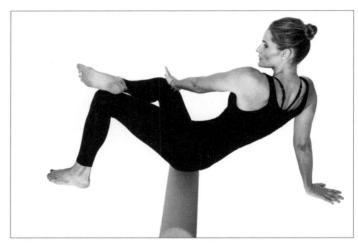

Kneeling Side Kicks

- Come to a kneeling position and place the roller to the right of your body. Reach your left arm up and exhale as you bend your body over to the right side until the palm of your right hand comes down to the roller at your side.
- Hold this position as you extend your left leg long and slightly in front of you.
- Inhale as you reach your left arm toward your right shin, keeping the roller stable. Exhale as you reach your left leg back and your left arm back in extension while bending the knee. Inhale as you reach your arm and leg forward. Exhale as you reach back.

Repeat this movement eight to ten times, then repeat on the other side.

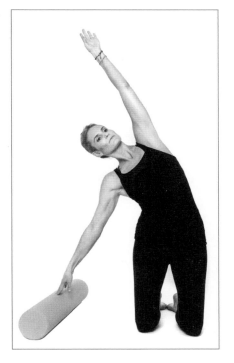

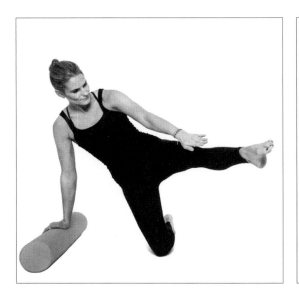

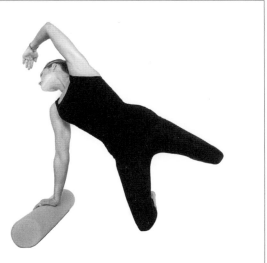

Roller-Supported Jackknife

- Lie down on your back on the mat, bend your knees, and place your feet down on the mat, hip width apart. Lift your hips up off the mat and slide the roller under your hips and sacrum, just above the tailbone. Lift your knees up directly over your hips and then slightly extend your legs straight up to the ceiling. Bend your elbows out to the side to anchor your upper body firmly on the mat and press your palms into the roller.
- Inhale as you lower your legs to a 45-degree angle, keeping your belly drawn in.
- Keeping your core, hamstrings, and arms active the entire time, exhale as you roll your spine and hips over your head until your legs are parallel to the floor.
- Exhale as you reach your legs up to a 45-degree angle.
- Inhale again as you begin to roll yourself back down with control, one vertebra at a time. Exhale to come all the way down, returning your hips and sacrum to the roller.

Repeat this movement eight times.

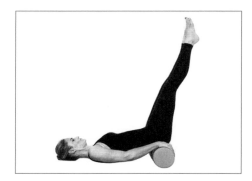
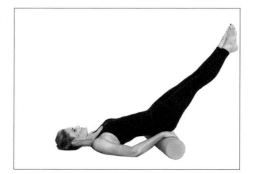
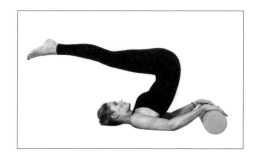
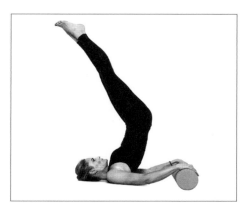

Physical Benefits

- Narrows and elongates the hips and upper thighs.
- Helps lift your core to stand taller and feel lighter.
- Brings more flexibility to the hips.
- Reduces tension in the hips.
- Sculpts more 3-D tone around the hips.
- Releases toxins stored in the hips.
- Reduces cellulite around the hips.

MOVEMENT REBOOT

Since we are elongating and freeing the hips in this session, take some time to tune in to how your hips move as you walk. Throughout the day today, take a moment to notice if your hips sway from side to side as you stride. This lateral motion of the hips is extremely important because it keeps energy flowing and helps to establish longer, leaner, more flexible hips and body. Also as you walk, take your hands to your sacrum to see how mobile your hips and pelvis are. Ideally, you will feel a nice, even side-to-side motion. If you don't feel that, adjust your walking until your hips fall into that back-and-forth rhythmic pattern. If you're not already walking like this, it might feel a little bit bizarre at first—but your entire body will thank you in the long run.

Adore Your Pelvic Floor/ Base of Core

Inner Thighs and Base of the Pelvis

Sleek and toned inner thighs and a strong core are every woman's dream. Little do people know that many times that annoying jiggle is caused by an overly tight and tense pelvic floor. Imagine a vertical line running down the center of your body from head to toe—that's your medial line. That's exactly what we're going to home in on today. You'll be releasing and strengthening the base of your core, which also releases and tones your inner thighs and the pelvic floor muscles. The end result is that you'll lift your entire core structure upward and create more balanced tone in your inner thighs, which lends itself to a taller, more balanced and youthful appearance.

Lateral Lunge

- Stand on your mat with your feet spread into a straddle position, about three to four feet apart. Stand the roller up vertically on the floor in front of you.
- Place your hands on top of the roller, with arms extended and spine straight.
- Inhale as you lean to the right, bending your right leg and straightening your left leg. Exhale as you hold the stretch.
- Repeat this motion on the other side.

Repeat this movement five times on each side.

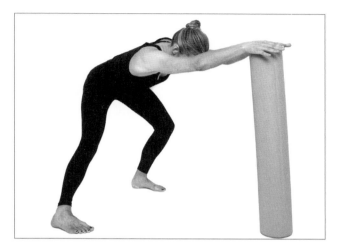

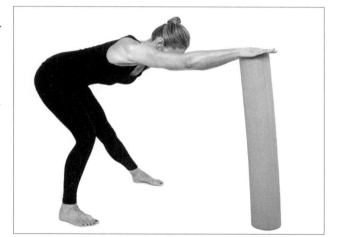

Inner Thigh Roll

- Come down to your forearms with your torso facing the mat, and place the roller under your right upper inner thigh. To do this, you will need to bend your right knee up and out to the side and place the foam roller up and under your groin.
- Taking care to keep your upper body square to the floor as you move, use your forearms and left leg to power the motion as you roll the roller down toward the knee (stopping just above it) and back up again.

Repeat this motion six to eight times on each side.

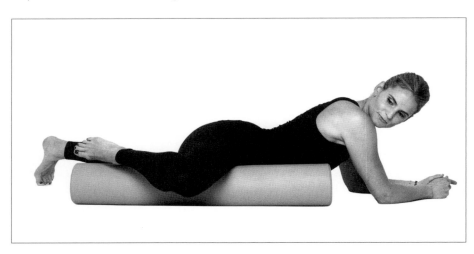

Sitz Bone Roll

- Place the roller on the mat and sit on it so that your sitz bones are directly on the roller.
- Extend your right leg long and roll the roller approximately two inches in each direction as you keep your breath smooth and long. This motion will reduce density where your adductors and hamstrings attach to your pelvis.

Continue this movement for thirty seconds, then switch to the other side.

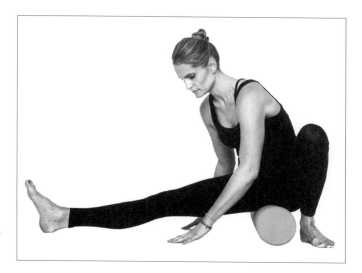

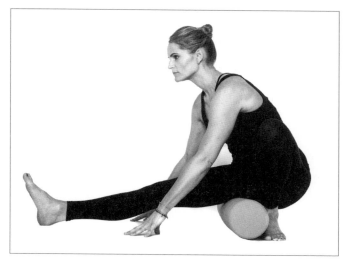

Side Kicks/Inner Thigh Lifts

• Bring your right hip down to the mat and place the roller under your right side at your waistline. Place your right elbow directly under your right shoulder joint. Bend your top knee and bring the heel of your top foot in front of you, with your knee facing up to the ceiling. Straighten your bottom leg.

• Inhale as you use your inner thigh to lift the lower leg, keeping your upper body and the roller stable.

• Exhale as you lower your bottom leg to the mat.

Repeat this motion eight times on each side.

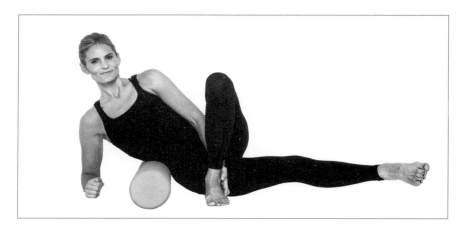

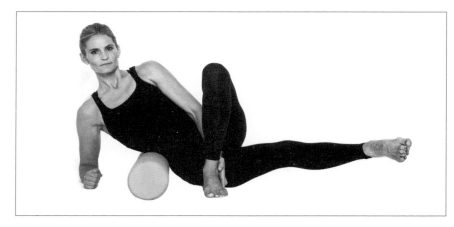

Roller Rx

Jumping Your Way to Pelvic Health

One out of every four women in the United States suffers from urinary incontinence, which is the involuntary loss of bladder control while sneezing, coughing, having sex, or laughing. Urinary problems in women, especially post-baby, are a huge epidemic. I've found that rebounding for five to ten minutes per day can have a dramatically positive impact on building healthy tone in the pelvic floor, repositioning the bladder, and helping to regulate minor incontinence by activating the pelvic floor while jumping. It's helpful to empty your bladder right before your jumping session (and even during, if necessary). Little by little, the tone will build back up. Your partner will thank you for activating these muscles!

Inverted Core Series

- Lie down on the mat and place the roller under your sacrum. Keeping your upper back and shoulders on the mat, elevate your waist in a bridge position while maintaining a neutral spine. Bring your knees over your hips and then extend your legs to about a 90-degree angle so they're pointing up to the ceiling. Place your hands on both sides of the outer edge of the roller to keep it stable throughout the exercise. Note that your spine should remain stable and neutral for the duration of this exercise.

- Inhale as you slowly lower your legs down toward your mat. Bring them down as low as you can without any sensation or arching in your lower back or shoulders.

- Exhale as you use your deep lower belly to draw your legs back up toward the ceiling to 90 degrees.

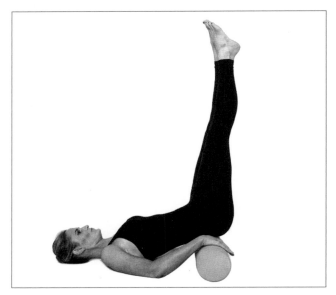

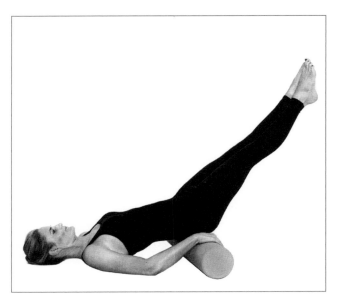

Repeat this movement eight to ten times.

Physical Benefits

• Improves sexual pleasure.

• Prevents and treats bladder issues.

• Strengthens and tones the base of the core.

• Helps your face look and feel calmer.

• Brings your body back to balance after childbirth.

MOVEMENT REBOOT

Chances are you ladies have heard of Kegels before. They are most commonly cited as a means of enhancing sexual pleasure (and good news—indeed, they do!). But aside from that, Kegels also connect us to our pelvic floor; they offer us a means of feeling the contrast between a relaxed and a tight pelvic floor. By identifying with that relaxed state, we learn to release the pelvic floor, which also relaxes and connects us to the base of our core and allows us to lengthen and lean out. Not only that, but with Kegels we also create a mind-body balance of control and surrender, effort and relaxation.

Without even realizing it, we hold a lot of tension in our pelvic floor. Think about how you react when you're in a stressful meeting or stuck in traffic. Do you clench your jaw or your butt? Both of these reactions are symptomatic of a tight pelvic floor.

Today try doing a few rounds of Kegels to experience the difference between a tight and a relaxed pelvic floor. To do this, imagine that you are trying to stop peeing midstream. Hold that motion as you inhale; then release as you exhale. Once you've familiarized yourself with both of those states, check in regularly for the rest of the day. Notice what your pelvic floor does when stress arises. Are you squeezing or holding tension? Whenever you notice this reaction, take a nice long exhale and release. Check in when you're walking, driving, or attending a meeting. Is there any amount of release and relaxation you can bring to the pelvic floor? When you *do* release that area, notice how your whole body changes—how you can move with more ease, and how other areas such as your jaw and tush relax as well. Ah, freedom.

Flat Belly Session

Deep Core and Psoas

It's time to stop hiding your glorious belly! The stomach is a serious area of concern for so many women. I can't tell you how often people ask me for tips to flatten their belly or reduce the post-baby pooch. Contrary to what many believe, doing thousands of crunches every day or running for miles won't earn you a flat belly. The trick is to release tension in the tummy, calm your nervous system, stand and move in alignment, and create length and balanced tone—*not* to tighten the abs. This sequence will help bring oxygenated blood to your belly, as well as flushing toxins and reducing density. As Daniel Bienenfeld, Hellerwork Structural Integration master trainer and practitioner and author of *Align for Life: Journey to Structural Integration,* says, we're going to "[empower] you with the awareness of your amazing psoas muscles, ultimately igniting your inner strength."

This sequence will draw your focus to the front of the spine, the belly, and the deepest core muscle, the psoas, to help align your spine, reorganize your core, and release you to the deepest muscles of your pelvis and core. You'll work on properly aligning the pelvis to its correct and neutral position, which will automatically flatten your belly, draw your organs in, and connect you to your powerful psoas muscles. You will look and feel taller and slimmer, not to mention enjoy improved digestion and abdominal organ function.

Psoas De-Bunch

• Lie on the mat faceup, with the roller placed under your sacrum. Bend one knee and draw it into your chest. Keep the other leg extended down on the mat in front of you, reaching long through the leg and pointing your toes.

• As you inhale, lift your extended leg two inches off the mat. Hold here for three slow, full breaths, allowing your hips to fully extend and elongate. After your third round of breath, exhale as you release your extended leg down to the mat, reaching through your flexed heel.

Repeat this movement eight to ten times on each side.

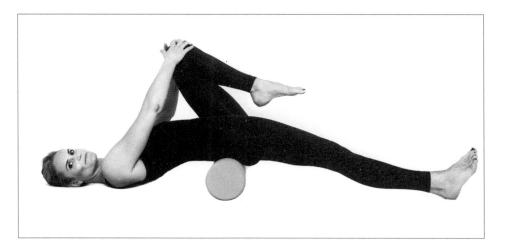

Psoas Backbend Twist

- Come down to your knees and place the roller directly behind you. Bring your right hand as close as you can get it to the middle of the roller behind you, and lift your left arm up to the ceiling. Lift your hips up and forward.
- Keeping the roller stable, inhale as you begin lowering your hips and your left arm down in front of you.
- Exhale as you press your hips forward and up, lift your deep core muscles up, and return to the starting position.

Repeat this motion eight times on each side.

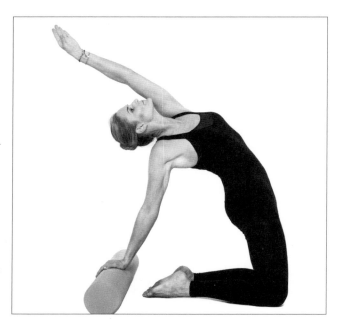

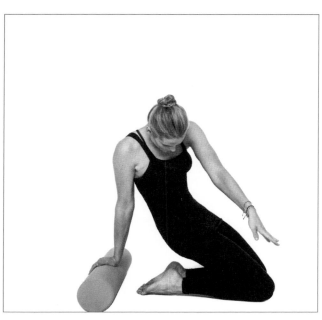

90-Degree Psoas Roll

- Come down to your forearms with the roller placed perpendicular under your left hip. Bend your left knee so that your heel is pointing toward the ceiling. Place your right inner knee and thigh parallel to the roller.
- Twist your body slightly to the right to expose your psoas, and roll up and down the attachment of your hip and psoas, keeping your breath smooth as you move. (Note that this is a very small and slow movement—you'll be rolling no more than two inches.)

Repeat this movement eight times, then repeat on the other side.

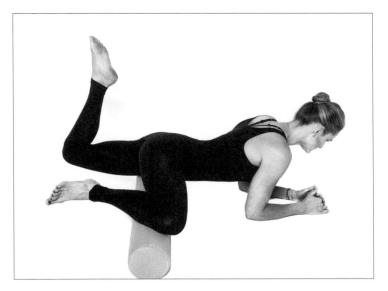

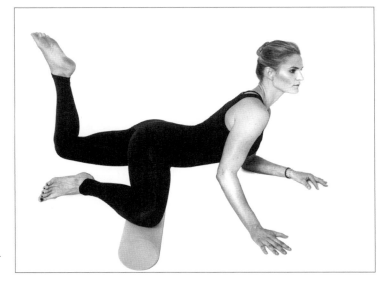

RESHAPE

Balancing Core Work

- Lie on the roller with a neutral spine, with the roller supporting you from head to tailbone. Place your forearms on either side of the roller to stabilize. Lift your legs with your knees bent at a 90-degree angle with your heels together and toes apart. Your knees should be shoulder-width apart.
- Lift your shoulder blades off the roller and curl up over your bra line, keeping a long neck.
- Keeping your curl engaged, inhale and extend your legs out to no lower than a 45-degree angle.
- Exhale as you bend knees back in while you maintain your curl.

Repeat this movement eight to ten times on each side, alternating sides.

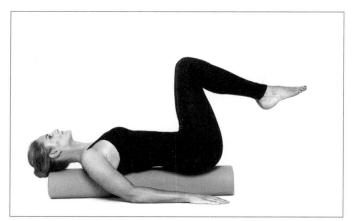

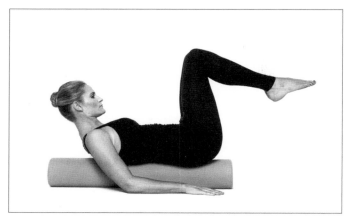

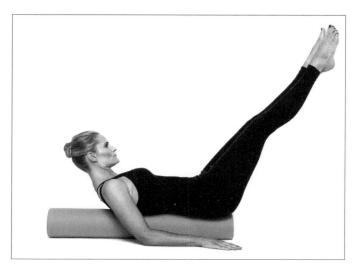

Rolling Lunge

- Stand on your right foot with your right knee slightly bent, and put the top of your left foot on the roller behind you with your back leg straight. Raise your arms directly overhead.
- Inhale as you bend your right knee, keeping the knee over the heel, and extend your left hip and leg back, pressing into the foam roller as it rolls up your shin until your right thigh is nearly parallel to the floor.
- Exhale as you use your deep core to pull yourself back up to the starting position.

Repeat this movement eight times on each side.

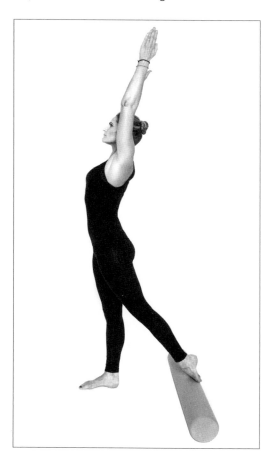
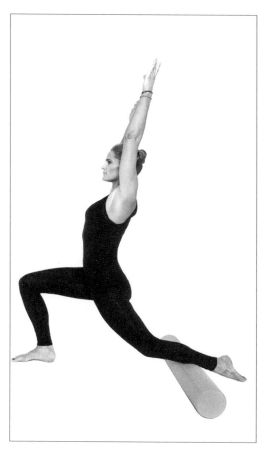

Physical Benefits

- Deepens your sense of leg movement from the core, rather than the hips.
- Balances the pelvis and aligns th pelvis, spine, and core so that they can move more freely.
- Flattens your belly.
- Promotes more conscious eating habits.
- Reduces lower back pain and tension.
- Makes steps longer and more fluid.
- Increases hip extension and builds longer, leaner hips.
- Enhances digestion, absorption, and elimination.
- Brings you more in touch with and makes you more aware of your organs.
- Helps you feel when you are full faster.

MOVEMENT REBOOT

As you walk today, pay attention to how it feels like your legs begin at the hip joints and notice how short your steps are. Now walk imagining that your legs begin just below your rib cage, at the point where your psoas starts. Notice how your stride is longer and your core and spine feel freer when you walk using your psoas. With every step you take, you are engaging the spine and core muscles, and your entire body is moving with grace and fluidity. Mindfully integrate a more expansive gait into your daily body movements.

DAY 9

Muffin Top Melting

Back of the Core

You are going to feel delicious after today's session. Not only will you melt away your muffin top, but you'll also work toward a more flexible, fluid, elongated, and decompressed spine. You know that wonderfully rubbery feeling you get after a massage? That's the same thing you'll achieve through today's sequence. You'll mobilize and tone your spinal muscles and the back of your legs, with a focus on releasing and strengthening the deep muscles of your back. Tuning in to these powerful intrinsic muscles will keep your spine erect for a taller, sleeker appearance. Looking good and feeling good—what more can you ask for?

Slinky Spine

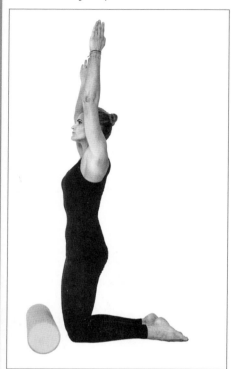

- Kneel, placing the roller a few inches in front of you. Inhale as you reach your arms up.
- Exhale as you round your spine down to roll into a kneeling forward fold that looks like an upside-down U. Be sure to soften your knees to help gently open the lower back.
- Inhale as you reach your spine into a full extension, chest down and sitz bones up; roll the roller up your forearms.
- Inhale to curl your tailbone under and pull your belly in as you roll yourself back up to the starting position like a Slinky.

Repeat this movement four times.

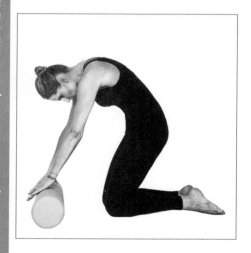

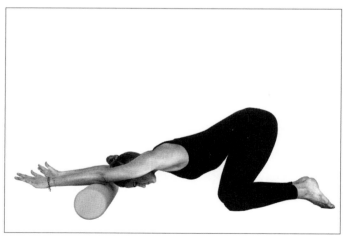

SMOOTH-OUT

Spinal Vertebrae Mobilization

- Place the roller under your midback at your bra line. Place your feet on the floor hip width apart, knees bent. Keep your hips planted on the mat for the duration of this exercise. Interlace your hands behind your head to support your head and neck.

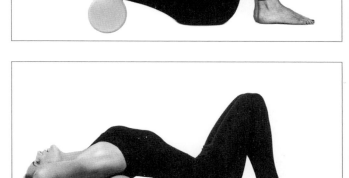

- Keeping the roller stable, inhale as you extend your upper back over the roller to mobilize your thoracic spine.
- Exhale as you curl back up.
- Next, push into your feet to move the roller up your spine one inch. Inhale as you extend and arch your back over the roller. Exhale as you curl back up. Keep going up your spine inch by inch until you have rolled all the way up to the top of your shoulders.
- Reverse your way back down your spine in the same manner until the roller reaches the bottom of your rib cage.

Repeat the entire process three times.

QL Roll

• Place the roller behind you.

• Come to a figure-four position with your left knee bent, right ankle crossed over your left thigh, right above the knee. Your forearms should be on the mat, palms on the roller, thumbs facing in. Lean your body to the right while feeling a subtle pressure on the right quadratus lumborum (QL), a lower back muscle between the bottom of your ribs and the top of your hips.

• Keeping the roller stable, press down into your foot while you inhale and curl your tailbone up; exhale and come back down.

Repeat this movement eight times on each side.

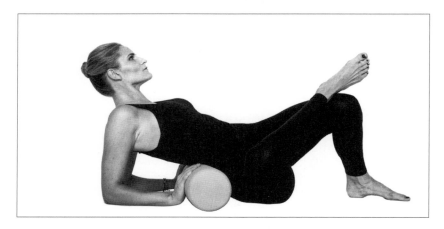

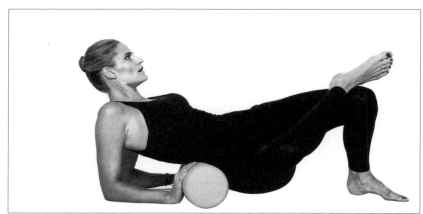

Rolling Swan

- Lie belly-down on the mat, with arms long in front of you and the roller placed just below your elbow joints, thumbs facing up. Reach your heels away from your heart to feel oppositional energy and decompress your spine.
- Inhale and roll the roller toward you, extending your spine and lifting your heart as you roll your shoulders back (taking care to keep your glutes relaxed the entire time so you don't jam your lower back while lifting up). Be sure to pull your abs up and in to support your back and elongate the front of your body.
- Exhale as you slowly resist on the way down, returning to the position you started in.

Repeat this movement eight times.

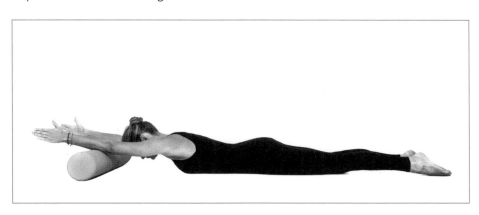

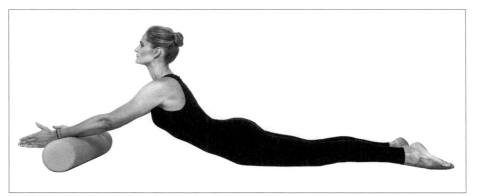

Roll Like a Ball

• Sit on the mat with your knees bent and bring the roller in front of your shins, holding on to either end of it with your hands. Relax your shoulders, broaden your back, deepen your abdominals, and make a balanced C-shaped curve of your spine from head to tail. Lift your feet off the mat and balance on or just behind your sitz bones.

• Inhale as you pull your lower abs in and let gravity roll you back to the top of your shoulders, smoothing out the tissue of your entire spine. Maintain the C-shape.

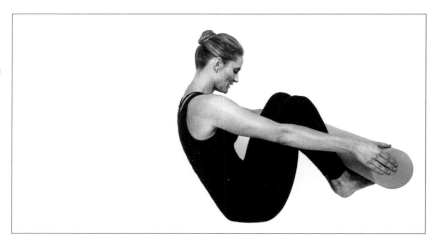

• Exhale as you return to the upright position and pause to balance, all the while keeping your belly scooped and your spine in a C-curve.

Repeat this movement eight times.

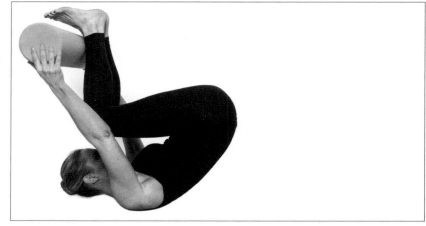

Physical Benefits

- Balances spine and spinal muscles.
- Elongates sides.
- Reduces muffin top.
- Brings more mobility to the spine.
- Provides the spine with more undulation.
- Decompresses the vertebrae.

MOVEMENT REBOOT

First things first: What does it mean to undulate your spine? Well, it's a natural pattern of moving our bodies fluidly through multiple joints in smooth, graceful, wave-like bends and curves, from front to back and side to side. We are all born with this ability, but most of our bodies have lost it due to aging and stress. Undulation of the spine requires the healthy and supple functioning of all of the core muscles along the spine. The undulation itself helps to nourish the spinal disks and ligaments, which is important for maintaining a supple and youthful spine. Maybe you've heard the old saying "You are only as young as your spine"? Well, it's true. And that's where undulation comes into play.

This simple but highly effective exercise can be done when you need a quick break at the office. On a chair, sit on your sitz bones. Let your spine sway from side to side like a willow in the wind. This will mobilize your vertebrae and make space for your spinal disks. Let the rest of your body relax and simply respond to this movement; take special care to release your neck. Next, try extending your spine forward to arch; then sit back on your sitz bones, turning your tail under to go into flexion. This simple movement will help bring more hydration and lubrication to your connective tissue while simultaneously giving you a boost of energy.

Elegant Neck

Collarbone, Neck, Jaw, and Head

Today you are going to lift up your head and neck for a longer, more graceful look. Now that you've spent the past nine days working through your entire body, you can finally release the head and neck, where we hold so much tension and do lots of processing. Throughout the following sequences, you'll bring awareness to the top of your core and free up any tension or excess stress. We're looking to restore a more vertical alignment to the neck and head by reducing the forward-leaning posture of the head that is so very common in this day and age. This session will also help you gain more freedom of movement in the head, neck, and jaw, and will restore tone and subtle strength and length in the neck, while relaxing the jaw and the face—all of which we tend to lose with age.

The neck is one of those areas of the body that often gives our age away, no matter how youthful or diligent we are otherwise. We'll combat this by doing some movements that expand and preserve elasticity in the neck, head, and jaw. Increasing flexibility and tone in the neck can help you look and *feel* years younger!

You'll sustain everything we learn today by discovering how to properly hold, properly align, and release tension in the head, neck, and face, all of which can dramatically help reduce stress, and rigidity. This awareness will help build subtle strength to improve your posture and help you look and feel more youthful and confident.

WARM-UP

Arms—Back Neck Rolls

- Come to a seated position on your roller and reach your arms behind you. Interlace your fingers and press your knuckles down toward the mat behind you.
- Inhale as you roll your head to the right; exhale as you roll it to the left.
- Next, imagine you have a pencil on your nose and are going to draw a circle. Take your head around in a full circular movement that lasts for an entire inhalation and exhalation. Repeat this movement in the reverse direction.

Repeat each movement eight times on each side and in each direction.

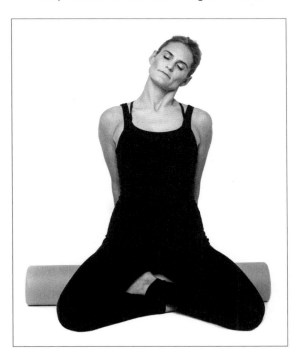
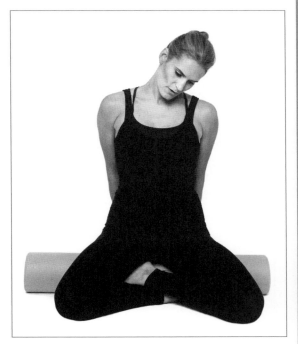

Neck Massage

- Lie down on your back and place the roller at the base of your skull, putting your hands on either end to stretch the arms and keep it steady.
- Inhale and turn your head to the left, feeling the roller gently massage your neck.
- Exhale as you come back to center.
- Inhale to fully rotate your neck to the right. Exhale as you return to center.

Repeat this movement eight times on each side.

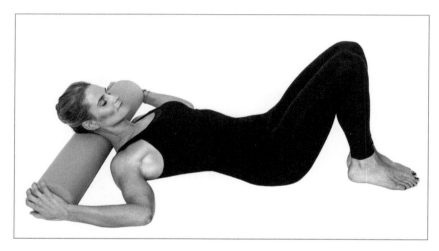

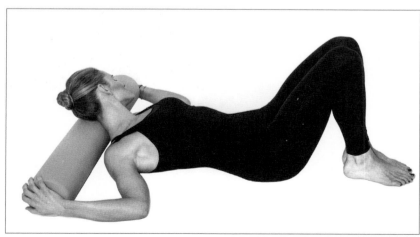

Collarbone Alignment

- Place the roller behind your upper back with your elbows bent and palms up. Bend your knees and plant your feet on the floor together.

- Exhale as you simultaneously lower your knees to the left and look to the right. Inhale to lift back to center and then exhale as you lower your knees to the right and look to the left. Inhale to lift back to center.

Repeat this movement eight times to each side.

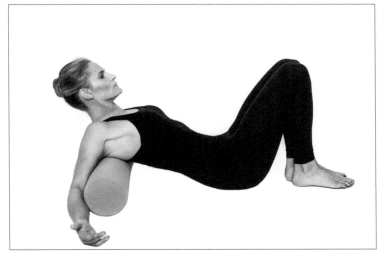

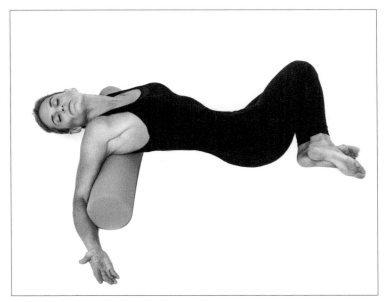

Rolling Mermaid Twist

- Place your right shin in front of you and your left shin out to the left side so that your knees are staggered. Place the roller to the right of you and put the palms of your hands on the roller. Reach and lift your sides and lift through the top of your head.

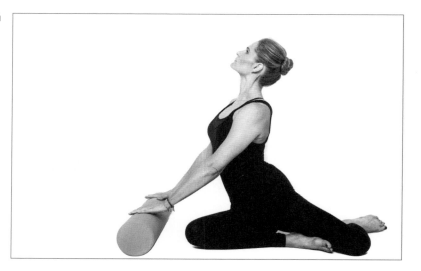

- Inhale as you roll the roller up your forearms to just below your elbows.

- Exhale as you roll back up to the starting position.

Repeat this movement five times, then repeat on the other side.

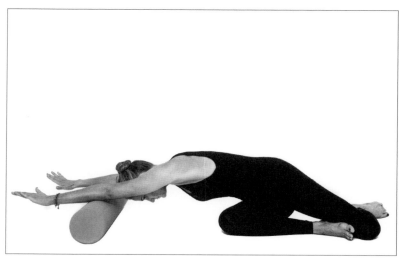

Starfish

- Come down to the mat and sit on your sitz bones. Place your right shin in front of you and your left shin out to the left side so that your knees are staggered. Place the roller to the right of you and place the palm of your right hand on the roller.
- Keeping the roller stable, lift your hips up and forward while you reach your left arm up and back, following your arm with your gaze and elongating the neck.
- Inhale as you start lowering your hips back down, simultaneously curling your chin and neck back down and circling your arm in front of you toward the roller.

Repeat this movement six times, then repeat on the other side.

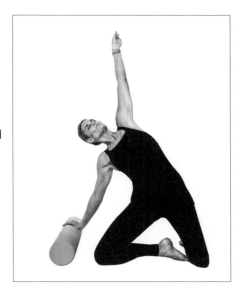

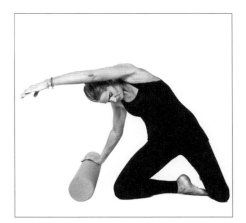

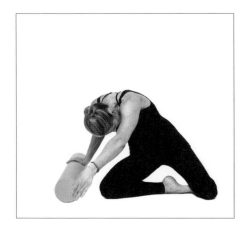

MOVEMENT REBOOT

While you're walking around today, tune in to and feel the way you hold your head. Notice if you feel any tension or rigidity in the muscles of your neck, face, head, and jaw. Are you clenching or tight in any of these areas?

Now imagine that your neck is a spring and your head is bobbing around like a bobblehead. See if you can allow your lower jawbone to become slack while you're walking or typing at your computer, even let your tongue relax away from th eroof of your mouth. I'm willing to bet that you'll feel an instant uptick in your mood when you do. And here's something to feel even happier about: Letting go in this way will help soften any wrinkles on your face. Finally, when you're at a point in your day where you're rushing around or stuck in your head, notice if you're leading with your neck or head like so many of us tend to do. Take a second to pause and bring yourself back to that bobblehead relaxed motion.

The body is an amazing machine. Even though adjustments like this may feel foreign at first, if you take the time to keep adjusting to this natural, clam-state, soon your brain will begin to create new neural pathways and healthier ways of responding to daily life that will keep you aligned and relaxed.

Aligned Life

DAYS 11–21

10 SERIES WITH A MIND-BODY FOCUS

We'll spend the second half of this program becoming more aware of the relationship between mind and body. The purpose of these movements is to integrate balance into your life by teaching you new ways of eliminating unhealthy habitual patterns in both the body and the mind. By learning new ways of using the body, you will be empowered to carry this renewed sense of self with you throughout your day and apply it to other areas of your life, even after you're done with the movement exercises. The questions asked of you in the introduction to each day are an opportunity for you to connect more deeply with your own inner wisdom, which will help you come into emotional alignment and release any emotional baggage that may be weighing you down. By changing your attitudes and perceptions about yourself and the world around you, you will discover new resources within. The daily Self-Care Second will help you unplug from the outer world and take a moment to tune in to your own inner compass.

Not only this, but we will also delve even more deeply into body awareness, which will allow us to enhance the fluidity, tone, and ease of motion that help develop a deeper awareness and appreciation of the body and its expression in the world.

Day of Restoration

Over the past ten days, you have established new movement patterns that will result in amazing physical benefits. By now you are likely beginning to have increased body and alignment awareness and a new appreciation for your miraculous body. You're probably also starting to feel how everything is connected, obtaining a real sense of your body in three-dimensional space, and gaining an understanding of its relationship to gravity, tension, and daily stress.

After all that focus, today is a day of rest. Your only job is to relax. Let's take some time to be present and to exist effortlessly in our bodies. We've all heard the preflight airplane spiel in which we're told to put on our own oxygen mask before helping others—even our children—in case of emergency. This is the perfect analogy for self-care. If we can't be there to take care of ourselves, we'll never truly be there for others.

We're beginning our discussion of self-care on a "rest day," but the truth of the matter is that some manner of self-care should be incorporated into your life each and every day—and *especially* on the days when you're *not* resting. Self-care doesn't have to be extravagant or expensive, and it doesn't have to be time-consuming. But it's vitally important to your own well-being, relationships, and reality. You will find that making time for self-care sends a message to you and your body that you are intrinsically valuable. When this message sinks in, you'll find yourself making decisions—even small ones—that support your true needs rather than the expectations of others. Doesn't that make you want to take a deep breath?

The key to enjoying and benefiting from self-care rituals is using all five senses to notice what it feels like when you are being good to you. Self-care time is a sort of playtime or recess from life, and it's all about your own enjoyment. It's so important that you take time to unplug, become present, escape the busyness of life, get off the hamster wheel, listen to your inner guide, and treat yourself daily. All of us unwind and rejuvenate in different ways, so my only instruction is to do so in the way that works best for you. Some suggestions include:

- Making a healthy smoothie
- Going to the farmers' market
- Pouring yourself a glass of wine at the end of the day
- Taking a salt bath (page 143)
- Meditating
- Listening to music
- Gardening
- Laughing
- Taking a nap
- Treating yourself to a pedicure

Whatever you choose to do for yourself, make that decision by asking yourself first, what you will *truly* enjoy, and second, what will be the most helpful in allowing you to relax and let go.

Looking Back to Move Forward

Part of treating yourself with care is acknowledging the good work you've done for yourself. This halfway point of the program is a good time to look back at what you've already accomplished over the course of the past ten days. Take five to ten minutes today to sit down and make a few notes about how you're feeling about your body. Are you more aware, more connected, and more in tune? Do you feel empowered with knowledge about your amazing body? Are you starting to see or feel physical benefits? How about emotional and mental ones? Note any physical, emotional, or mental changes (big or small!) you've noticed since beginning this program.

Connecting to Your Inspiration

Chest, Shoulders, and Arms

Now that you have worked on physically opening up the chest, ribs, diaphragm, shoulders, arms, and lungs while learning how to stand taller, you can look more deeply into how this area of the body affects you on an emotional level. You will, of course, continue to emphasize physicality and breath. But starting today I will ask you to think of breath not only as a means of inhaling oxygen but also as a primary method of filling yourself with life force and inspiration and of letting go and releasing stress. Be sure to keep your breathing expansive throughout these moves to ingrain this new, more layered and meaningful pattern of breath into your daily life to the point where it becomes second nature. (For more about breath, try out the umbrella breathing described on page 27.)

While you're doing these moves, ask yourself: *What truly inspires me? What really takes my breath away? And, contrastingly, what depresses and brings me down?* Today and every day for the remainder of this 10 Series, I strongly recommend recording your answers in a journal for future inspiration and a record of how far you've gotten at the end of this program.

Arm Circles

- Lie on the roller the long way, so that your entire spine is supported from head to tailbone. Reach your arms out to the side in a T-shape with the palms of your hands facing up to open and expand the chest.

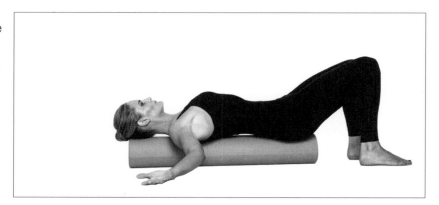

- Inhale deeply expanding your lungs as you reach your arms up overhead while keeping them parallel to the floor.

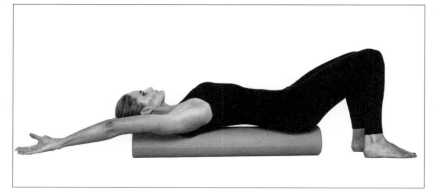

- Exhale as you draw your arms up to the ceiling and back down by your hips.

Repeat this movement eight times.

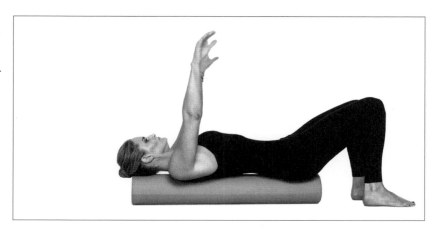

Roll Out the Kinks

- Lie on the mat with the roller placed under your back at the bra line, leaning your midback over the roller. Gently interlace your fingers behind your head to support your head and neck.
- Using your feet to drive the movement, inhale as you roll up to massage the upper back and shoulder blades, stopping at the top of the shoulder blades.
- Exhale as you roll and massage down the spine, stopping at the bottom of your rib cage. Be careful *not* to roll back and forth on the lower back because it can create too much pressure or force on your disks and vertebrae.

Repeat this movement eight to ten times.

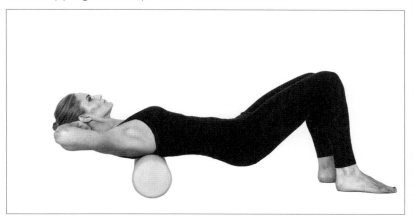

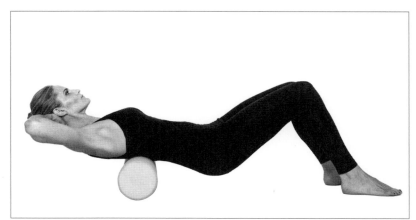

Diaphragm Release with Organ Twist

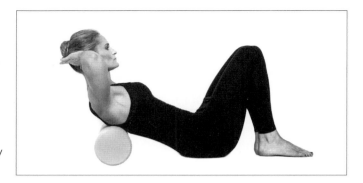

- Lie on the mat with the roller placed under your back at the bra line. Gently interlace your fingers behind your head to support your head and neck.

- Inhale as you arch your thoracic spine (or middle to upper back) over the roller.

- Exhale as you twist your legs and hips to the left, squeezing and wringing out your organs.

- Inhale to bring your knees to center and repeat this motion to the other side.

Repeat this movement eight to ten times on each side, alternating sides.

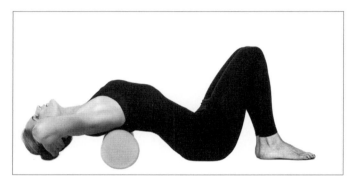

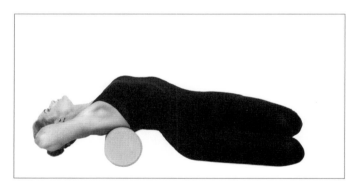

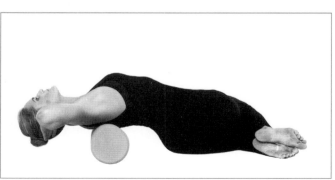

RESHAPE

Rolling Swan with Arm Pulls

- Lie belly-down on the mat, with arms long in front of you and the roller placed just below your elbow joints, thumbs facing up. Reach your heels away from your heart to feel oppositional energy and decompress your spine.
- Inhale and roll the roller toward you, extending your spine and lifting your heart as you roll your shoulders back (taking care to keep your glutes relaxed the entire time so you don't jam your lower back while lifting up). Be sure to pull your abs in and up to support your back and elongate the front of your body.

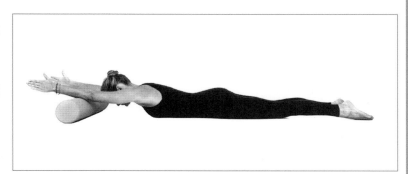

- Remaining in this suspended position and keeping your shoulders drawn down, exhale as you pull your elbows back toward you. Continue to remain suspended as you inhale to straighten your arms. Repeat this arm pull six times.

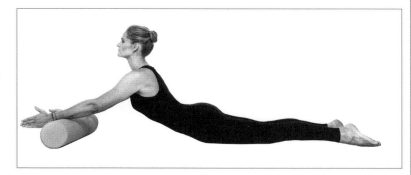

- Exhale again as you slowly resist on the way down, returning to the starting position.

Repeat this movement eight times.

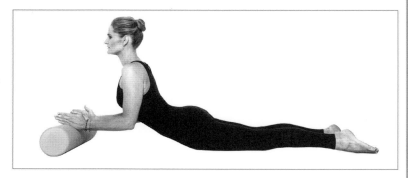

Rollover with Arm Presses

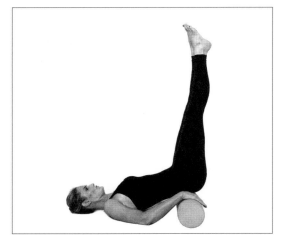

- Lie down on the mat with the roller placed just above your sacrum so that your hips are on the roller, with legs extended toward the ceiling. Place your palms on top of the roller, with your elbows slightly bent to open your shoulders and chest and engage your triceps.
- Inhale to lower your legs down to a 45-degree angle, keeping your core strong to avoid loading your lower back.
- Exhale and start rolling over into an inverted U-shape, keeping your body suspended and abs and hamstrings engaged.
- Inhale again as you slowly roll your body halfway down, decompressing your spine and activating your triceps.
- Exhale as you return to the starting position.

Repeat this movement six times.

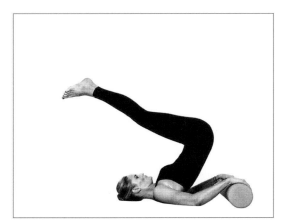

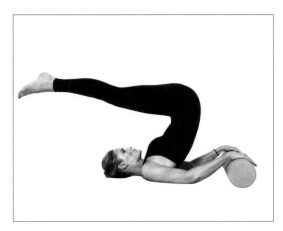

Roller Rx: Shape Your Shoulders

Remaining in the active part of this movement at both the halfway down and halfway up positions will open the front of the shoulders and shape the muscles on the back of your arms into a more proper alignment.

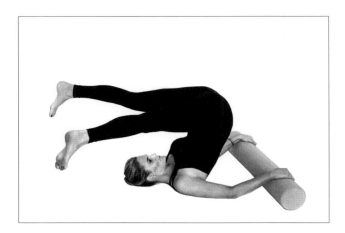

Reverse Triceps Dip

- Sit down on the mat and place the roller behind you. Place your palms firmly down on the roller shoulder-width apart, with your pinkie fingers facing out. Press your feet into the mat to lift your tush off the floor. Open your chest, lengthen your neck, and draw your shoulders back.
- Bend your knees up toward the ceiling so that your heels are directly under your knees. Plant your feet firmly on the floor hip width apart, lift your hips up, and straighten your arms.
- Keeping the roller stable, your core engaged, and your chest open to avoid hunching, inhale as you slowly bend your elbows behind you.
- Exhale as you press up to a soft elbow, taking care to avoid locking the elbow joints.

Repeat this movement ten times.

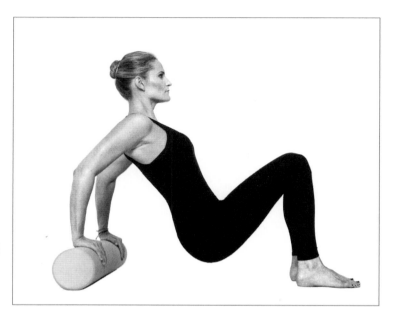

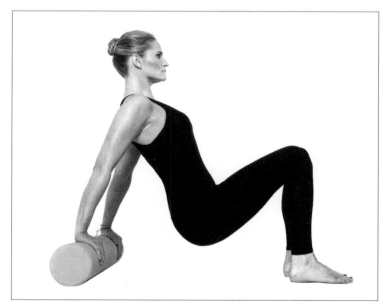

Emotional Benefits

- Improves the ability to deal with stress.
- Encourages the heart to be more open.
- Improves confidence.
- Takes "the weight of the world" off your shoulders.
- Helps curate a deeper sense of self.
- Helps connect you to what inspires *you*.

SELF-CARE SECOND

Create a Happy List! Take a few minutes out of your day to unplug from all modes of technology and make a list of all the things that make you happy. Then make a list of all the things you do every day, compare the lists, and adjust accordingly. Keep the list somewhere you can easily access it at all times and make it a goal to incorporate these items from your Happy List into your daily life on a regular basis.

Find Your Foundation

Feet, Ankles, and Lower Legs

Beyond just realigning and reshaping the lower body, this session relates to the idea of standing on your own two feet. Think of someone you know who is down-to-earth, centered, calm, and grounded. Now think of someone who is an unstable, scattered, chaotic drama queen floating through life. Who would you rather hang out with? Thought so. Grounded people tend to be more charismatic, organized, present, practical, successful, and realistic. When people are grounded and present in their physical bodies, they are generally more emotionally grounded as well, and naturally draw more of that same energy into their lives. The most successful and efficient people have mastered grounding and are thus able to slow down, make a conscious choice to live life to the fullest, be present, avoid distractions and drama, and let go of or altogether avoid toxic people, things, and activities that waste precious time.

As you go about your day from here, pay attention to your feet as you walk and feel all twenty-six joints doing their work to keep you grounded. Let your back foot be the driving force that moves you forward.

While doing today's moves, ask yourself: *How grounded do I feel in the world financially, emotionally, physically, and spiritually? When stressful situations arise, do I become overly dramatic or do I stay calm, knowing life is like riding a wave—sometimes it will knock you over? Do I look at uncomfortable times in life as growth spurts or am I concerned only about what others think or say in the moment?*

Toe Tendon/Joint Mobilization

• Come down to a deep squat position. Shift the roller under your mid-upper shins and keep your toes curled forward, with toes spread wide and heels reaching back so that your feet are really stretched out. Keep your elbows soft and place your hands shoulder-width apart on the mat. Keep your shoulders drawn down for the duration of the exercise.

• Use your feet to roll forward and back, stretching your feet and rolling your shins.

Repeat this movement eight times.

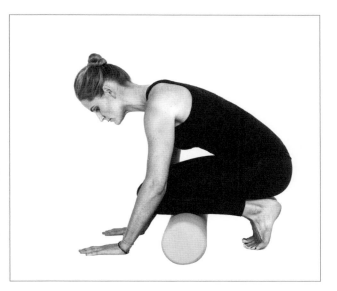

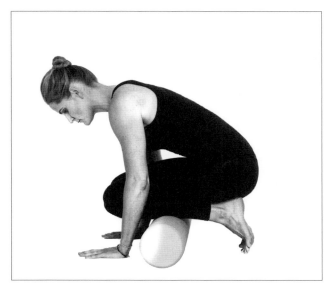

SMOOTH-OUT

Tennis Ball Arch Roll

- Stand next to a wall or sturdy chair where you can steady yourself and place a tennis ball under the heel of your left foot.
- Roll the ball back and forth from your heel to your toes for 30 seconds; then switch feet. Start with a softer pressure for your first round. Then gradually apply a bit more weight as you go deeper into the fascia and mobilize your feet.

Repeat this movement four times on each side, alternating sides.

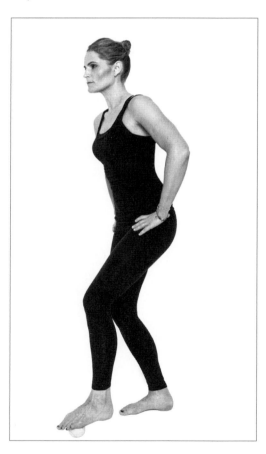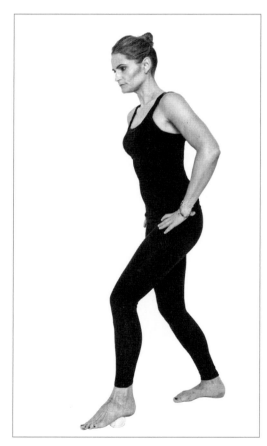

Kneeling Lunge Shin Roll

- Come to a kneeling lunge on your mat, beginning with your right leg forward and bent at a 90-degree angle. Place the roller just below the kneecap of your left leg. Place your hands slightly in front of your shoulders on either side of your foot.

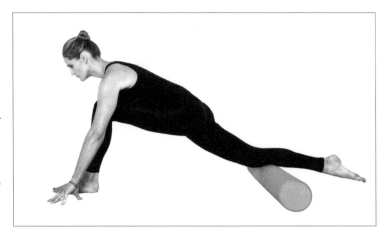

- Inhale as you ground through your front foot and pull yourself forward, straightening your back leg as the roller rolls down your shin.
- Exhale as you return to the starting position.

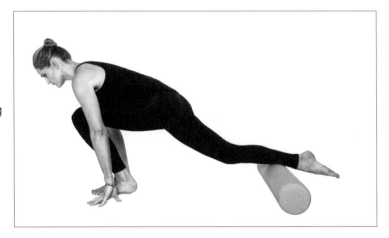

Repeat this movement eight to ten times per leg.

Calf Roll with Rotations

- Sit on your mat with your legs close together and the roller placed under both of your calves, right below the knee joint. Place your hands palms-down on the floor a few inches out from either side of your hips, fingers pointing outward. Press down into your hands to lift your bottom off the mat, keeping your calves balanced on the roller. Make sure to draw your shoulders down and back to avoid hunching.

- Continue pressing your hands down and engage your core, exhaling as you slowly drive your body weight forward so that the roller stops right above the ankle.

- After you've finished rolling down the center of your calves, internally rotate your feet (turn them inward) and repeat this rolling motion, this time rolling through the inner part of the calf.

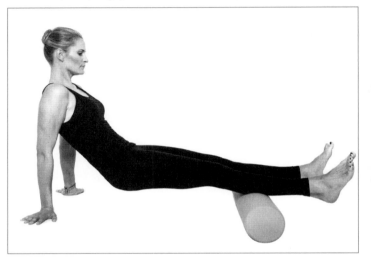

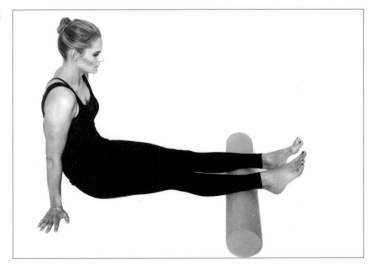

- Externally rotate the feet (turn them outward) and roll, this time along the outer part of the calves.
- Return to parallel and release yourself back to the floor.

Repeat this movement eight times per variation.

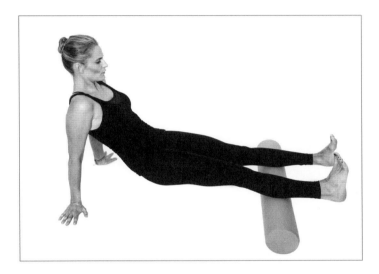

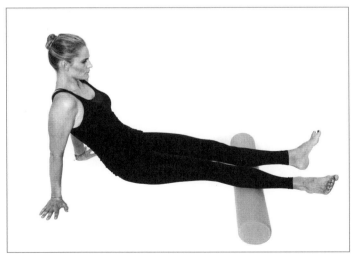

Rolling Leg Pull Front

• Place the roller under your hands and come to a push-up or plank position, keeping your entire core and arms engaged. Reach your heels back, spreading your toes and really stretching the feet and arches.

• Inhale as you shift your weight forward onto your toes while lifting your heels as the roller moves forward and your abs kick in even more.

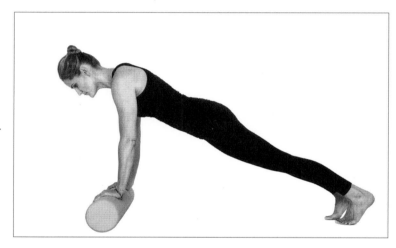

• Exhale as you reach your heels back to stretch your feet and activate your core while using your abs and feet to press the roller back.

Repeat this movement ten times.

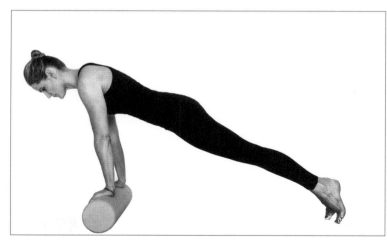

Rolling Bridge Heel Pulls

- Lie on your back, bend your knees, and place the roller under the balls of your feet. Reach your arms long by your sides.

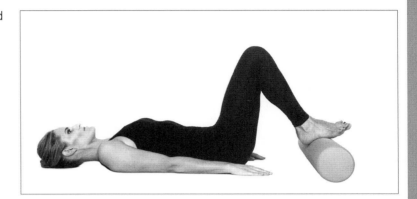

- Inhale as you start to roll your spine up one vertebra at a time and exhale all the way up until you're in a bridge position.

- Inhale again as you pull the roller an inch toward you and then exhale as you push the roller back one inch. Repeat this movement as a pulsation eight times.

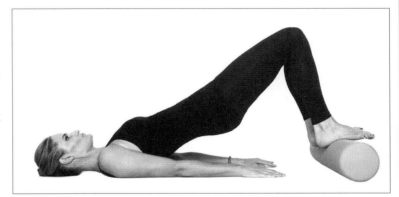

- Exhale as you roll your spine down one vertebra at a time and extend your legs in front of you.

Repeat the pulling portion of this movement eight times.

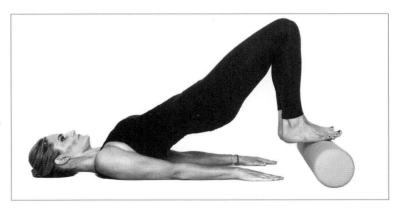

Emotional Benefits

- Helps to feel more grounded and calm.
- Generates a feeling of peace in the present moment.
- Increases body-mind awareness.
- Improves the ability to deal with stress as it arises.
- Boosts self-esteem.
- Helps r educe anxiety.

SELF-CARE SECOND

Walking barefoot in the grass or on the beach can help you connect to your center and to the earth. "Earthing," or going barefoot, helps ground you and nourish your body with electromagnetic energy directly through the soles of your feet. Research shows that going barefoot has the ability to calm and center you, and even reduces tension and inflammation. It may also help you sleep better, reduce stress and pain, and increase immunity.

DAY 14

Fluid Forward Motion

Legs

As the workhorses of the body, the legs are associated with how we progress through life. Think of all the expressions we have that relate to the legs: "Stand up for yourself." "Stand your ground." "She doesn't have a leg to stand on." All of these catchphrases reference our foundation in some way, shape, or form, which is precisely what our legs do—they simultaneously give us a foundation and move us forward in life. Our legs take us where we want to go . . . but where do we want to go?

As you're moving forward today, ask yourself the following questions: *How easy or hard is it for me to stand up for myself? To make decisions? To move forward?* Notice how you actually move and whether you take short steps instead of long, graceful, and courageous ones. Once you've observed your movement patterns, notice how they align with your own sense of foundation and forward movement.

Standing Stability

- Come to stand on the foam roller with the arches of your feet at the center of the roller, aligning your body's center of gravity over your feet. Find your neutral spine and maintain a slight soft bend in your knees as you balance on the roller.
- For stability and support, hold on to a nearby wall, chair, or counter.

Continue this balance work for one to two minutes, getting back on the roller when (and if!) you lose your balance.

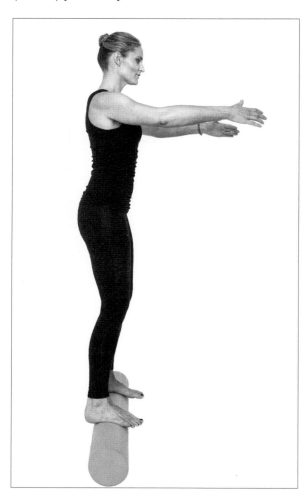

SMOOTH-OUT

Back of Thigh Roll

- Sit on your mat with the roller under your hamstrings, right above the knee joint. Place your hands on the mat behind you, with fingertips slightly turned out. Press your hands into the mat to lift your bottom off the floor and engage your core.
- Keep your shoulders back and inhale as you roll the roller up the back of your thighs.
- Exhale as you roll back down to the starting position.

Repeat this movement eight to ten times.

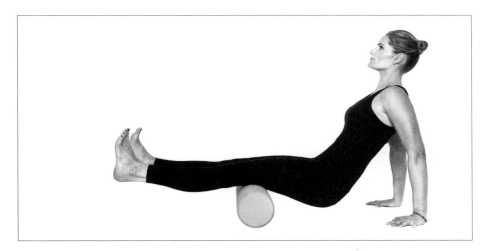

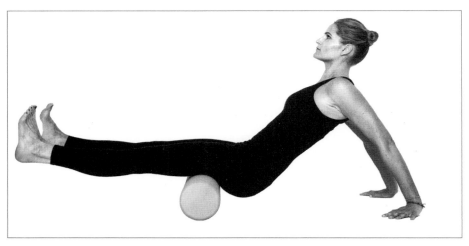

Front of Thigh Roll

- Place the roller above the knees. Bring your elbows to the mat about two inches behind your shoulders and make fists. Engage your core to prop yourself up and protect your lower back.
- Using your arms and core, exhale as you pull yourself forward as the roller rolls up the front of your thighs.
- Inhale as you press the roller down to just above the front of your knees.

Repeat this movement eight to ten times.

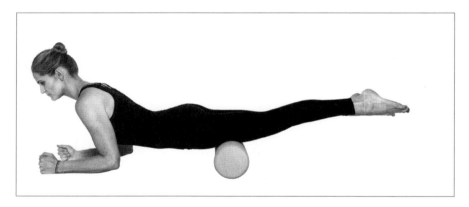

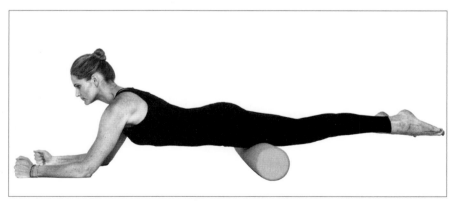

Thigh Stretch Twist

- Kneel on the mat with your knees hip width apart, big toes together. Bring the roller over your head, placing a hand on either side of it. Keep your shoulders down and chest open. Establish a neutral spine (see the box on page 20) and maintain a stable spine and pelvis throughout this exercise.
- As you inhale, begin hinging back from your knee joints. Engage your inner thighs and pull your belly in and up to keep the weight off your knees and press your shinds down into the floor.
- Exhale and twist your entire body to the right.
- Inhale back to center and exhale to the left.
- Inhale to return to center and exhale back up to the starting position.

Repeat this movement five times on each side, alternating sides.

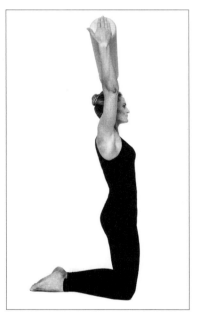
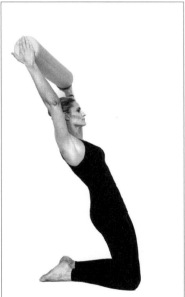
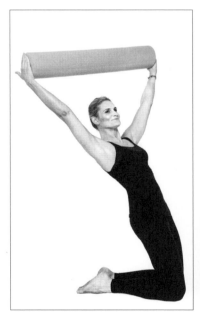

Rolling Lunge

- Stand on your right foot with your right knee slightly bent, and put the top of your left foot on the foam roller behind you with your back leg straight. Raise your arms directly overhead.
- Inhale as you bend your right knee, keeping the knee over the heel, and extend your left hip and leg back, pressing into the foam roller as it rolls up your shin until your right thigh is nearly parallel to the floor.
- Exhale as you use your deep core to pull yourself back up to the starting position.

Repeat this movement eight to ten times, then repeat on the other side.

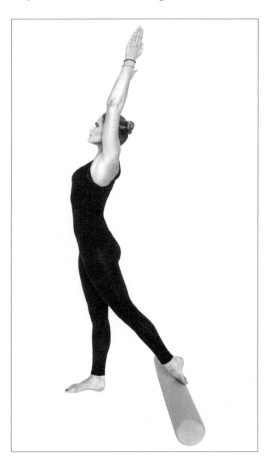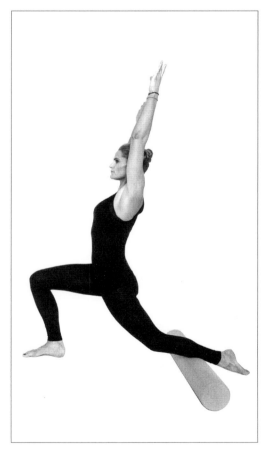

Emotional Benefits

- Connects you to what you stand for.
- Increases your courage to move forward.
- Releases emotional baggage held in the legs.

SELF-CARE SECOND

Say goodbye to toxins, cellulite, and dull skin with dry body brushing! This is one of the easiest and least expensive ways to stimulate your lymphatic system (which serves as the circulatory system's waste removal system) and to flush toxins, especially from the legs. Doing this also stimulates the connective tissue attached to the capillaries sitting under your skin, which improves circulation through the body.

To brush, I like to use a sisal natural fiber body brush by Mio. Start at the feet and brush your way up your inner and outer legs to your hips, waist, tummy, backs of the arms, chest, back, and shoulders, always moving the brush in the direction of your heart. Avoid brushing your face or other sensitive pink parts, as well as any areas of the body.

Once you've brushed your entire body, jump in the shower and rinse the dead skin away with some hydrotherapy. Alternate between the hottest and coolest temperatures you can tolerate to stimulate blood circulation and boost metabolism. Continue to dry-brush your entire body for a few minutes every day to compound these benefits.

Expansion vs. Compression

Waist, Lower Back, and Sides

Beyond just realigning and reshaping the sides of your body and reducing tension in the upper body, this session is a physical representation of how you emotionally expand versus contract or compress. You will continue working on creating a more uplifted and grounded self that will allow you to more easily expand when you need to, whether from a physical, emotional, mental, or spiritual standpoint.

Here's a simple little test to gauge your body's current ability to expand. Notice the weight of your arms. Do they feel light? If so, that means you are overworking your shoulders and upper back muscles, compressing your waist and lungs, and tightening your shoulders, ribs, and upper back. Release your shoulders and feel your arms become heavy. Now notice how the sides of your body feel. Is there any tension? Make a concerted effort to release this tension, allowing your arms to become heavy, your shoulders to relax, and your breath to expand. The goal is to have heavy, long arms, with relaxed shoulders and an elongated and strong ballerina neck.

Just as we bring tension and heaviness into our bodies, we also bring it into our emotional lives. Take a quick survey of your current emotional state. *Where do I feel compressed and where do I feel expanded?* Often emotions like anger or frustration make us feel tense and compressed, whereas more positive feelings like compassion and happiness make us feel expansive and connected. This session will allow the body to move toward its desires and open up to aligned manifestation.

Rotating Wood Chopper

- Stand in a straddle position, with your feet about five feet apart. Hold on to either edge of the roller and reach your arms overhead.
- Inhale and begin bending to the right.
- When you have bent about halfway, rotate your torso down toward the right side of the mat. Be sure to keep your knees soft so you don't stress your back or knee joints.
- Gently swing the roller over to the left, using your waist to draw your upper body over to the left side, and then curl back up to stand.

Repeat this movement three times, then repeat on the other side.

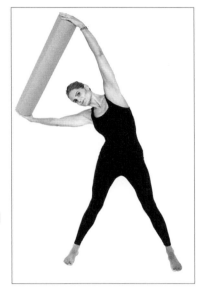
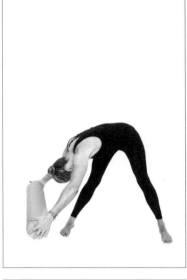
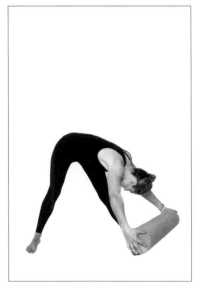
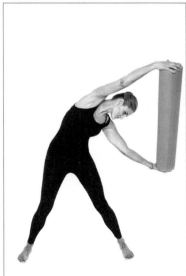

SMOOTH-OUT

12th-Rib Roll

- Bring your left hip down to the mat and place the roller at your waistline (below your left lower ribs and above your left hip). Stack your left elbow under your left shoulder and bring your left forearm to the mat so it's running parallel to the roller. Keep your left hip on the mat, bend your right knee, and ground your right foot in front of your left knee.

- Inhale as you gently rock forward, leaning and twisting your upper body toward the roller.

- Exhale as you roll your ribs back to center.

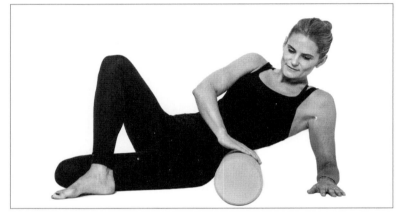

Repeat this movement six times on each side, alternating sides.

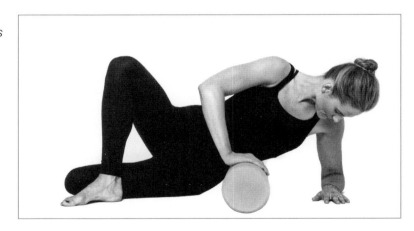

Figure Four

- Sit on the roller and reach your right arm behind you with your right hand on the mat, thumb out to the side. Cross your right ankle over your left knee in a figure four position. Press your left hand down into your right inner thigh.
- Shift your weight slightly over to the left hip/glute area and roll back and forth a few inches in each direction.
- Next, roll in circles to help increase circulation and blood flow and to reduce congestion.

Repeat this movement on the other side.

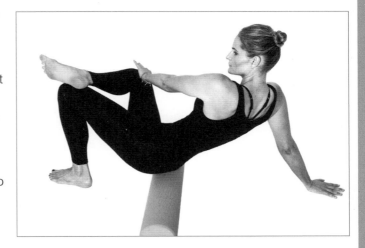

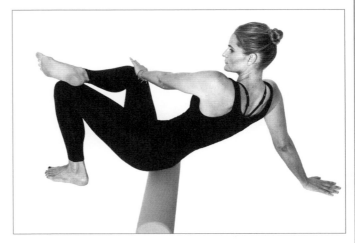

Outer Thigh Roll

- Lie down on your right side, placing the roller under the upper outside of your right thigh. Bend your left knee and cross your left leg over your right, placing your left foot flat on the floor in front of your right knee. Bring your right forearm down to the mat to ground you.
- Use your left foot and right forearm to roll the length of your iliotibial band (IT band) along the roller from your hip all the way down to just above your knee joint. (The IT band is the thick line of fascia that runs along the outside of your body, from your pelvis all the way down to just below your knee.) As you get closer to your knee, you may feel more tenderness, so be prepared to use your left arm and foot to ease the pressure. The more weight you bear in your foot, the less you will place on your IT band.

Repeat this motion eight times, then repeat on the other side.

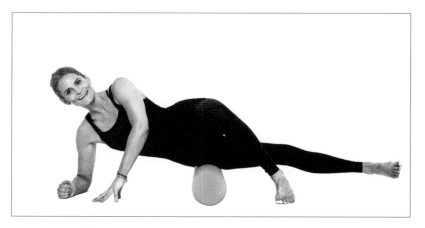

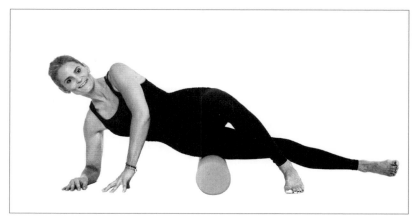

Hourglass with Arm Twist

- Place the roller under your left leg, just above the left anklebone, and cross your right leg over your left. Place your left elbow directly under your left shoulder, with your forearm flat on the floor and fingers spread; reach your right arm up and slightly back. Press down into your left leg and forearm, using this traction to lift your side body (or "hourglass") off the floor, taking care to keep the roller stable as you lift.

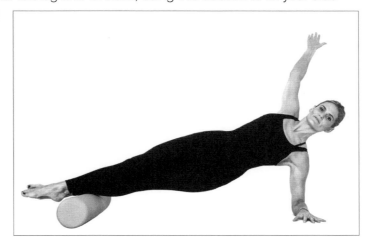

- Initiate the move with an inhale; exhale as you rotate your torso toward the left and reach your right arm under you to "thread the needle" while keeping your side body lifted. Follow your arm with your gaze by tucking your chin.
- Inhale as you lift your right arm back up to the starting position, again following it with your gaze as you move.

Repeat this movement eight to ten times, then repeat on the other side.

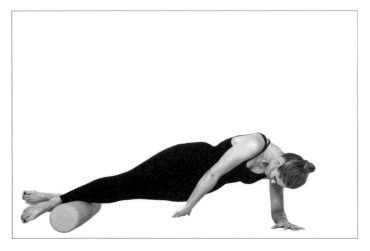

Roller Twist on Hip

- Lie on your right hip with your spine running parallel to the side of your mat and your legs hinged at a 45-degree angle toward the right front corner of the mat. Place the roller slightly below your right elbow joint.
- Inhale and gently press down into the roller to start rolling it to just above your wrist (this will tone your triceps and lats), while simultaneously lifting both legs up and rolling slightly to the left while balancing on your right tush and hip.

- Exhale at the top and hold while continuing to balance with the roller above your wrist.

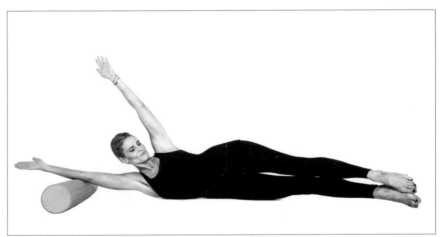

- Inhale slowly to start reaching long as you come down, and exhale all the way down to the mat as the roller returns to its starting position right below your elbow joint.

Repeat this movement eight times, then repeat on the other side.

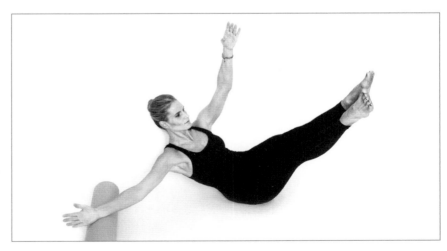

Emotional Benefits

- Helps you assert yourself in a relaxed manner.
- Provides a greater sense of ease when it comes to expanding or reaching out to others.
- Increases confidence.
- Enhances ability to deal with stress.
- Helps you feel more connected to others.

SELF-CARE SECOND

Reach out and hug it out. Science says that at least eight 20-second hugs a day will secrete the love drug, increase self-esteem, and decrease feelings of loneliness. Today hug someone you love for a full twenty seconds. The power of touch between humans can secrete one of the most important happy chemicals: oxytocin. Oxytocin helps calm your nervous system, reduce cravings, and decrease inflammation. It even helps you heal faster. Embracing for twenty seconds or more a few times a day can help you feel bonded and more positive, lower your blood pressure, and even boost your overall health. So go find someone to hug and spread the good vibes!

Stability Session

Glutes

We all love a strong booty, right? The tush is incredibly important for stability and agility, and it protects your knees and spine. Not to mention, it always looks amazing with some added lift and tone! Strong, toned, supple glutes are integral to the proper functioning and support of your legs, pelvis, and spine. When your tush is strong, toned, and flexible, the rest of your body doesn't have to work so hard to exist in gravity. When you value these muscles for the physical integrity they give you, you can start to feel more stable on the inside, too.

One of the definitions of the word *stability* I came across while writing this book is "the quality or state of someone who is emotionally or mentally healthy." Simple enough, right? (Or seemingly so, at least.) If you ask me, this is exactly what we should all strive for. From a mind-body alignment standpoint, having a strong and stable body helps you feel like you can deal with more, and stay calm and steadfast in the process of doing so. While you're doing these moves today, ask yourself: *How stable do I feel when the s#*t hits the fan? How resilient am I in response to drama and unexpected daily life experiences? What actions can I take to bring a sense of stability to those areas of my life that may feel shaky or unstable?*

Single-Leg Squat Kick

- Stand with your feet hip width apart and reach your arms out to the side, with palms down.
- Inhale as you lean into your right foot and lift and reach your left foot up off the mat.
- Exhale as you bend your right knee and come back to center, returning your left foot to the mat.

Repeat this movement ten times per side, alternating sides.

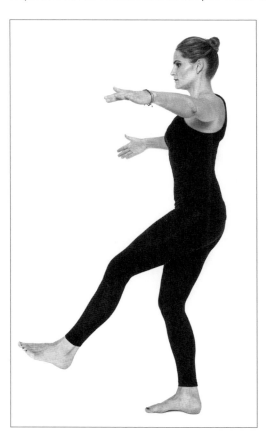
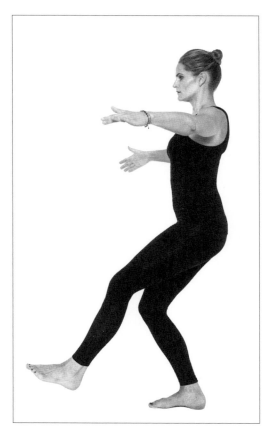

Glute Roll

- Sit down on your mat with the roller placed beneath your tush. Place your hands behind you on the mat. Bring your knees and feet together and lift your heels up so only your toes are touching the mat.

- Lean to the left side of your tush (including your knees), and roll from the inside to the outside of your tush so that you are massaging the entire side of the booty from the sacrum to the greater trochanter bones of the outer hip.

Complete this movement on each side for about thirty seconds per side.

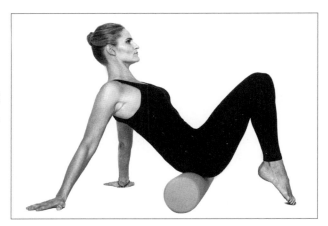

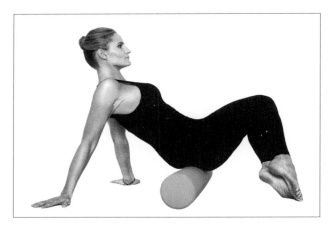

Figure Four Circular Roll

- Sit on the roller and cross your right leg over your left knee to form a figure four.
- Lean to the right so the pressure of the roller hits all of your glute, and roll in a circular motion around your tush, forward and back.

Repeat this movement eight times on each side, alternating sides.

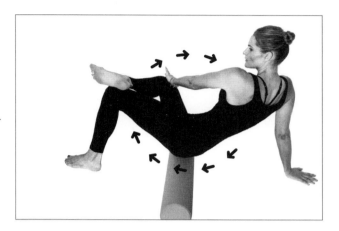

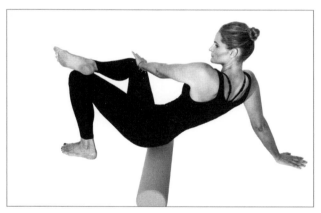

Roller Bridge Walk

• Lie on your back, reaching your arms long by your side, with your knees bent and feet placed on the mat hip width apart, about a foot away from your tush. Place the foam roller under the arches of your feet. Engaging your glutes, hamstrings, and core, press into your arms as you lift your hips up toward the ceiling so that your body forms a straight diagonal line from your knees and your shoulders.

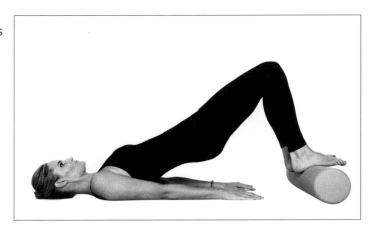

• Keeping your right knee bent, inhale as you lift your right foot and stabilize the roller with your left foot.

• Exhale as you return your right foot to the roller. Repeat the exercise with your left leg.

Repeat this movement eight times each side, alternating sides.

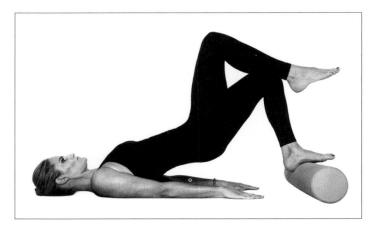

Kneeling Side Crab

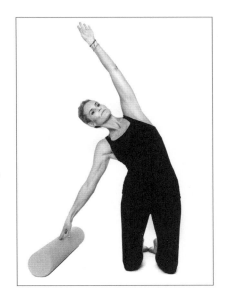

- Come to a kneeling position and place the roller to the right of your body. Stretch your left hand up toward the ceiling and exhale as you bend your entire body over to the right until the palm of your right hand comes down to the roller at your side.
- Hold this position as you bend your left arm behind your head, reach your left leg out to the side, and bend the knee to tone your outer tush. Inhale as you lift your left knee up to the ceiling while keeping your upper body, hips, and the roller stable.
- Exhale as you lower your top knee down, keeping the foot and ankle stable.

Repeat this movement eight times, then repeat on the other side.

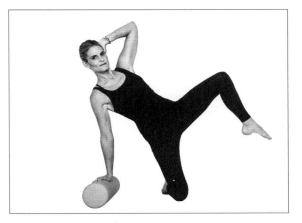

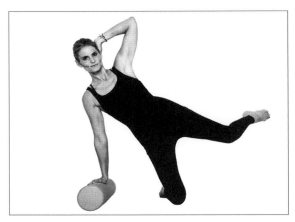

Emotional Benefits

- Increases confidence and connection to your body.
- Increases emotional stability and steadiness, which leads to greater success in all areas of life.
- Provides overall feelings of strength and inner support.
- Creates a greater sense of calm and balance.

SELF-CARE SECOND

Rebounding, or jumping on a trampoline, for five to ten minutes per day can be a great way to tone your tush, release stress, and increase energy and oxygenation in the tissue and blood. As I mentioned on page 12, research shows that rebounding is more effective for cardiovascular health and fat-burning than running. Plus, it's a fun, effective, low-impact, multidimensional form of movement that increases bone density and helps improve digestion and elimination. It also stimulates the lymphatic system, which bolsters immunity and circulation, and decreases cellulite, and lifts the booty. My favorite rebounder is the Bellicon, which you can find at laurenroxburgh.com.

Emotions in Motion

Hips

By now you know that if something is bothering you mentally or emotionally, it's likely to show up in your body—and especially in your hips. Since these emotions are a form of energy, when they are not released from the body, they become stuck and can turn into thickness, heaviness, tightness, and pain. I bet you've had the experience of feeling like you have a physical weight on your body when something weighs on your heart or mind, right? That's exactly the sort of experience I'm talking about. The good news is that the physical manifestation of emotional and mental pain is resolvable. Not only that, but there's also a beautiful chicken-and-egg effect, wherein resolving the physical manifestation of these issues also helps alleviate the emotional and mental discomfort of them. That's exactly what you'll be working on today.

The following moves will help you connect with whatever stored or blocked energy you're holding in your hips. They will bring this energy to the surface, cleanse it from your cells and tissues, and even help release it from your subconscious. While doing these moves, ask yourself: *What am I carrying? Do I have any unresolved resentment, anger, fear, or sadness?* Whatever you identify, let it go and enjoy the moment.

Standing Hip Circles

- Stand with your feet hip width apart, a tall neutral spine, and soft knees.
- Imagine that you are using your hips to draw large circles on a piece of paper. Inhale as you shift your hips over to the right and then circle them to the front.
- Exhale as you slide your hips to the left and finish by circling them to the back. The movement should be fluid and smooth throughout.

Repeat this movement eight to ten times, in both directions, moving in a fluid circle.

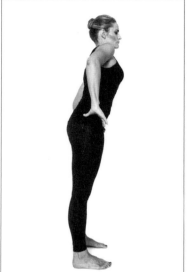 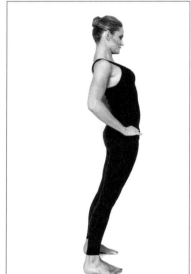

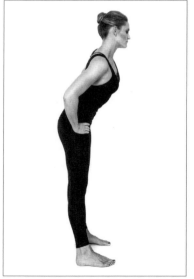 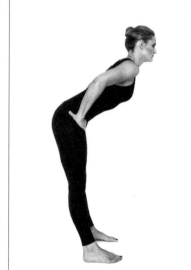

SMOOTH-OUT

Internal and External TFL Roll

- Place the area right above the bony part of your right hip and below your pelvis on the roller, targeting the tensor fasciae latae (TFL), a muscle that runs from the hip to the top of the pelvis. You will not have to roll much with this move as it covers a small surface area. Cross your left leg over your right, grounding down through your left foot.
- Inhale and exhale long and smooth as you use your left foot to create motion and roll up and down this small area eight to ten times.
- Internally rotate your foot and knee to roll the outer side of your TFL, again eight to ten times.
- Externally rotate your feet and knees to roll the more medial side of your TFL, again for eight to ten times.

Repeat each of the three variations of this movement eight to ten times.

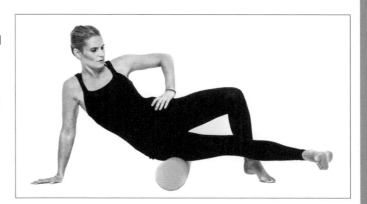
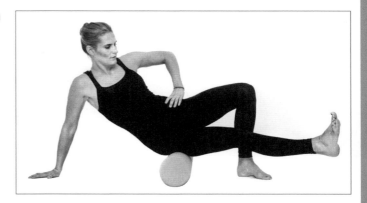
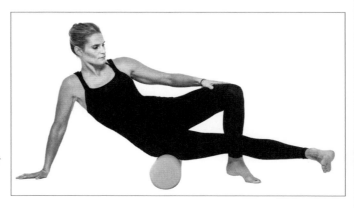

Front of Hip Roll

- Lie facedown on the mat and place the roller under your left thigh. Prop yourself up so that you are supporting your weight with your left forearm and right palm.
- Roll your weight slightly over to the left. Inhale as you roll the few inches along the front of your upper thigh to your hip, and exhale as you roll back down to the upper thigh. Repeat this movement eight times; then repeat on the other side.

Repeat this movement eight times, then repeat on alternate side.

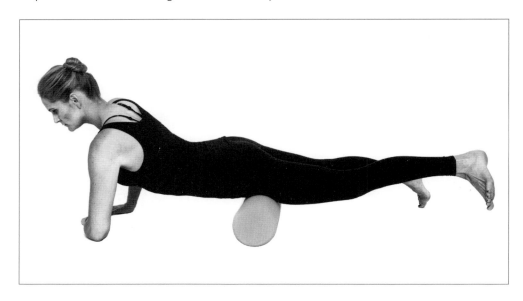

RESHAPE

Roller CanCan Balance

- Sit on the roller with your arms reaching behind you, palms planted on the mat, and fingers pointed out to the sides. Keeping the roller stable, lift your knees up over your hips and engage your abs.
- Inhale as you roll your hips and knees over to the right, so that you're balancing on the roller with your right hip.
- Exhale and extend your legs out to a 45-degree angle. Keeping your core connected.
- Inhale as you bend your knees back and turn so that your left hip is now balanced on the roller, repeating this motion from there.

Repeat this movement six times on each side, alternating sides.

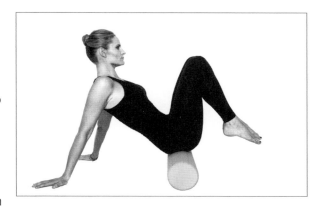

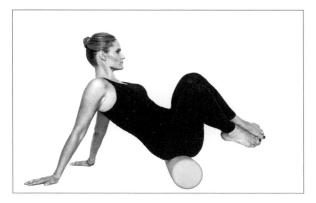

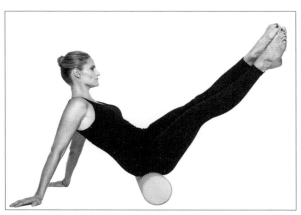

Crisscross Backbend

- Sit up tall with your ankles crossed, knees wide. Place the roller about six inches behind you and press your palms into the roller, thumbs out to the side.
- Inhale as you press your palms into the roller to lift up and press your pubic bone forward, gazing up as you lift through your chest.
- Exhale as you release back down to the starting position.

Repeat this movement eight to ten times.Switch the leg cross and repeat five times on each side.

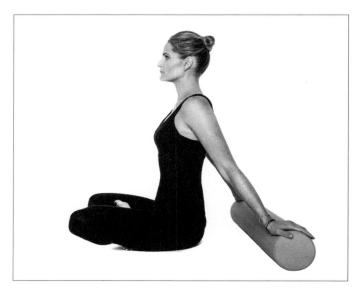

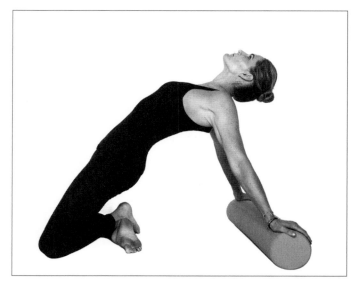

Emotional Benefits

- Releases toxic emotions and fear.
- Releases sadness.
- Releases anger and resentment.
- Fosters a sense of peace.
- Breeds a greater sense of joy.

SELF-CARE SECOND

A Himalayan salt bath is a rejuvenating, detoxifying, therapeutic, and relaxing at-home spa treatment for both body and mind. These salts are naturally rich in eighty-five trace elements found in the human body that nourish and replenish your skin and connective tissue. They also help draw out toxins, reduce soreness and tension, energetically cleanse the body, and remineralize tissues.

To prepare your bath, fill the bathtub with water and add one to two cups of Dead Sea or Pink Himalayan salts (I love Herbivore Botanicals Calm Dead Sea Bath Salts). Once the salt has dissolved into the water, soak in the tub for twenty minutes. Some soothing music and candles while bathing really enhance the experience! Don't rinse when you're finished bathing, and pat yourself dry. Relax, hydrate, and rest after the bath. You will sleep so deeply.

DAY 18

Connecting to Your Base and Roots

Pelvis

In many cultures, it's widely believed that the base of your core—or your root—is the place from which life force energy is drawn. By creating balance in your body and in your life, you are more able to feel safe, calm, and secure in the world around you. Daily life and all the tasks that are expected of you start to become effortless and more fun. Stress levels plummet, and doubts and fears disappear as you begin to feel yourself easily moving with the flow of life. When you find this natural flow, the world and the universe work with you.

Finding peace with your pelvic floor and hips allows you to deeply connect with your own authentic power in all areas of life. It's amazing how releasing the tight, rigid, physical blockage of energy that builds up at the base of the pelvis and hips frees up both your body and your life to transform in sometimes miraculous ways. With this ultimate body-mind connection and newfound physical freedom and strength comes a more joyful, loving, fluid life experience. You are able to accept and draw into your life what you truly desire, whether it's love, health, a fit body, money, career advancement, or anything else.

It's not what happens to you in life; it's how you deal with it. The exciting revelation of the sequence that follows is that stress is a reaction and you can control how you react. It's truly empowering! Some things to think about today: *How do I deal with stress as it arises? When do I allow myself to surrender in life?* Challenge yourself to really release and go with the flow during this sequence and see if you can bring that same energy into the rest of your day.

Sexy Cat

- Bring the roller in front of you and place your forearms on it, right below the elbow joints. Reach your sitz bones up and your chest down, feel your sitz bones opening like a flower blooming.
- Keeping the roller stable, inhale as you lean your hips over to the left.
- Exhale as you lean your hips over to the right.

Repeat this movement six times on each side, alternating directions.

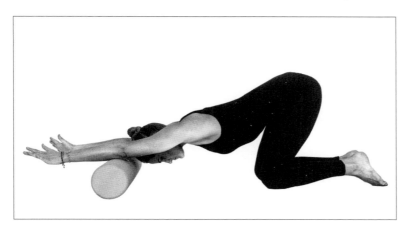

Pigeon Inner Thigh Roll

• Place the roller about a foot in front of you and come down to your knees. Bring your right leg in front of the roller so that your right calf is parallel to the roller, and lean forward into a pigeon hip stretch, so that the roller is now at the inner edge of your sitz bone. Use your front foot to keep the roller stable and lift up into a tall spine. Keep your left leg long and straight back behind the roller.

• Breathing steadily, slowly roll front and back to smooth out the inner thigh and pelvic floor attachment.

Repeat this movement eight times on each side, alternating sides.

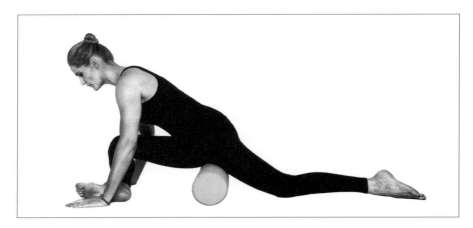

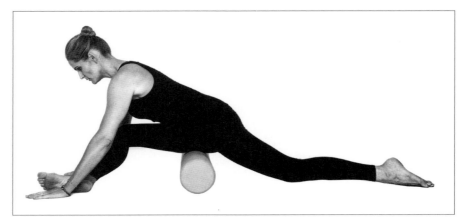

Goddess Pose Roll

• Place the roller under your hips, with your feet together and knees wide. Keep your belly engaged to prevent overarching your lower back. Come down to your forearms with your belly facing the mat.
• Exhale as you roll all the way down to your inner knees.
• Inhale as you roll up to your pubic bone attachment.

Repeat this movement eight times.

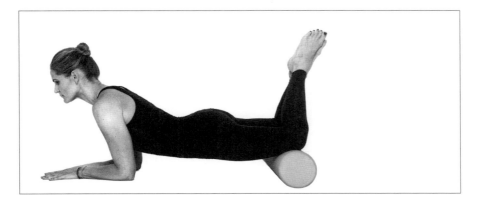

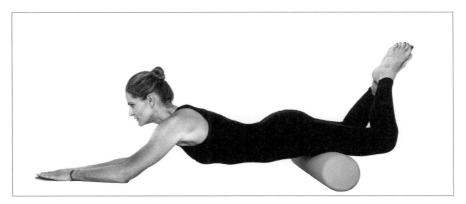

Seated Single-Leg Circle

- Sit on the roller and reach your arms behind you, chest and heart open, legs stretched in front of you and the back of your heels resting on the mat. Plant your palms down on the mat with fingers facing outward.
- Lift your right leg to a 45-degree angle. Keeping your breath smooth and your belly engaged, move your leg in a clockwise direction to make six slow, controlled circles. Repeat this movement six times on the left side.
- Lift your right leg so that it is elevated from the mat and repeat this same motion six times, but this time in a counterclockwise direction. Repeat this movement six times on the left side.

Repeat this movement six times on each side and in each direction, alternating sides.

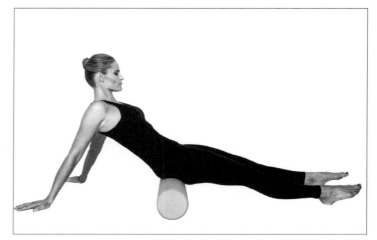

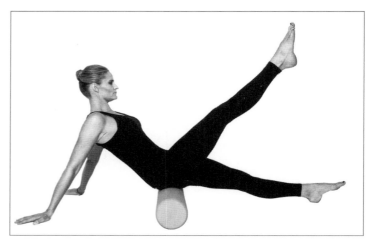

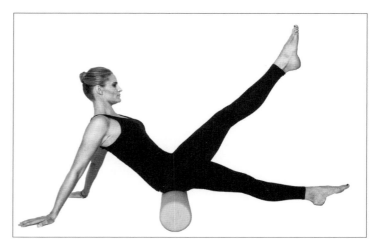

Inner Thigh Cross

- Sit on the roller and reach your arms behind you, legs stretched in front of you. Plant your palms down on the mat with fingers facing outward. Keeping your core engaged, lift both of your legs up to a 45-degree angle, heels together, toes apart.

- Inhale and exhale to lower your legs down a few inches.

- Continue to breathe slowly and steadily as you cross one leg over the other, alternating legs ten times.

Repeat this movement ten times.

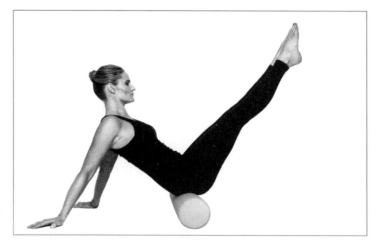

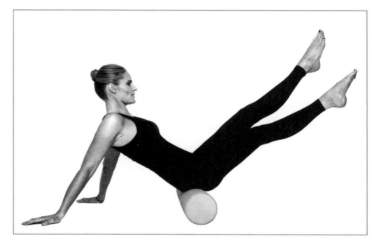

Emotional Benefits

- Boosts self-esteem.
- Makes you feel sexier.
- Teaches the balance of control versus surrender.
- Creates a greater sense of connection for your base.
- Generates more charisma.
- Supplies a sense of ease and grace in your body.
- Helps the body deal with stress more efficiently.
- Results in a greater sense of ease.

SELF-CARE SECOND

Have sex! Having sex is fun and it's great for your body, mind, and spirit—not to mention the fact that it truly helps bring you into the present moment. This is especially true during the moment of orgasm, when your body and mind both go off the grid. Sex chemically elevates mood and reduces depression, forsters connections and orgasms trigger a rush of endorphins and human growth hormones, while also reducing cortisol levels. Some studies say that people who have frequent sex look dramat-ically younger—up to *twelve years younger than their actual age*, in fact. So go ahead! Get it on.

Listen to Your Gut

Deep Core/Psoas

Did you know that we actually have brain cells in our gut, which phys-ically supports the idea of "gut instincts"? Yes, that's a real thing. This session will help you tune in to your gut feelings and connect to the visceral reaction that occurs before your mind takes over a situation. Science associates these feelings with brain cells in the gut or the "second brain" that send signals to the nervous system.

Our guts tend to shut down and become rigid in response to the fast, rigid ways of the world today. This area tightens up when we are under stress or over-worked, which results in losing touch with our true feelings and insightful intu-ition. This is a huge inhibitor to daily life because the body provides powerful information about our health, our decisions, other people, our surroundings, and ongoing situations. This information helps us create a positive environment for ourselves and limits our contact with toxic people and situations.

Throughout the day today, notice how your emotions relate to tension in your body, particularly in your gut and belly. *As emotions come up, breathe into your gut and feel and connect to your emotions as fully as you can. How does this feel?* Notice what happens in your body.

Psoas Rolling Lunge Twist

- Stand on your right foot with your right knee slightly bent, and put the top of your left foot on the roller behind you with your back leg straight. Raise your arms directly overhead.
- Inhale as you bend your right knee, keeping the knee over the heel, and extend your left hip and leg back, pressing into the foam roller as it rolls up your shin until your right thigh is nearly parallel to the floor.
- Exhale as you twist your body and arms to the right to stretch the psoas.
- Inhale to unwind back to center, and exhale to return to the starting position.

Repeat this movement eight times, then repeat on the other side.

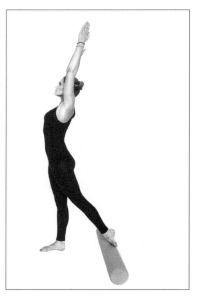 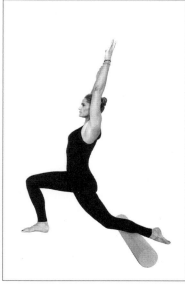 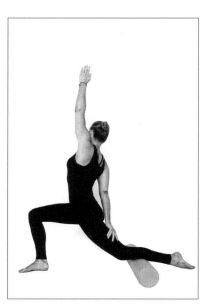

90-Degree Psoas Roll

- Come down to your forearms with the roller placed perpendicular under your left hip. Bend your left knee so that your heel is pointing toward the ceiling. Place your right inner knee and thigh parallel to the roller.

- Twist your body slightly to the right to expose your psoas, and roll up and down the attachment of your hip and psoas, keeping your breath smooth as you move. (Note that this is a very small movement—you'll be rolling no more than two inches.)

Repeat this movement eight times, then repeat on the other side.

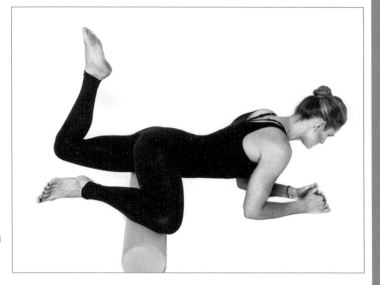

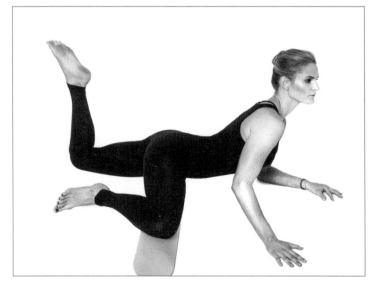

Rolling Shell

- Bring the roller right below your knee joint, legs together and extended, toes pointed. Place your hands on the mat shoulder-width apart and stack your shoulders directly above your wrists. Stabilize your shoulders by imagining there is a skewer through your shoulder joints to keep you from rocking back and forth.

- Inhale and start rolling the roller toward you while lifting your core and rounding your spine into flexion; take a full exhale to pull the roller all the way in while your hips lift, scooping your belly and sucking your tummy in.

- Inhale as you resist while slowly lowering back down; exhale to come all the way back to the starting position.

Repeat this movement eight to ten times.

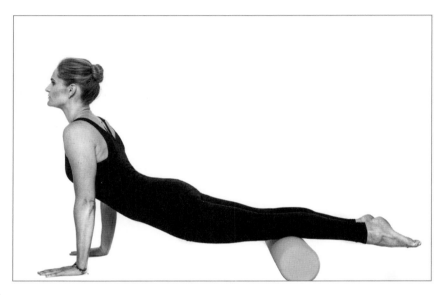

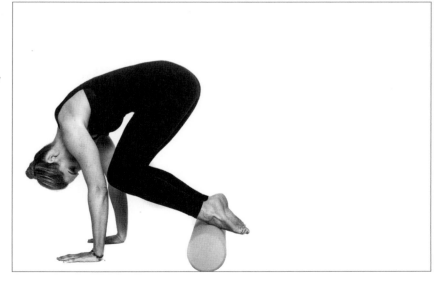

Advanced Grasshopper

- Place your lower thighs (right above your kneecaps) on the roller and your hands directly under your shoulders, fingers pointing forward. Inhale to bring your spine into extension, looking straight ahead.

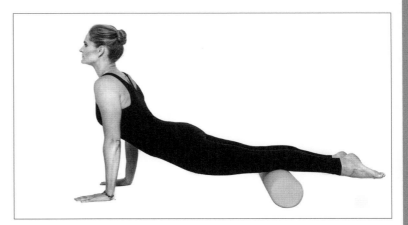

- Exhale and bend your elbows to lower down, hovering over the mat.
- While hovering, inhale and bend your knees, bringing your heels toward your tush.
- Exhale and extend your legs.
- Inhale and straighten your arms and lift back up; exhale and hold before beginning the next rep.

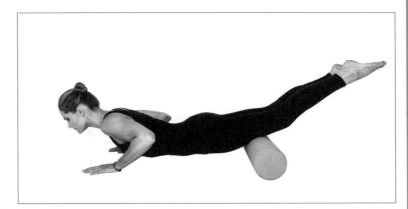

Repeat this movement eight to ten times.

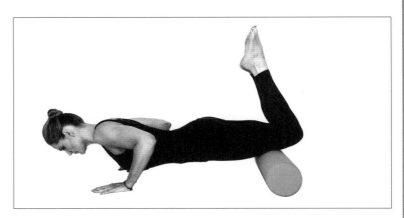

Emotional Benefits

- Builds the courage to follow your gut instincts.
- Helps reduce toxic energies in your life.
- Reconnects you with yourself.
- Helps you become more compassionate with yourself and others.

SELF-CARE SECOND

Nothing is more likely to bring you into the moment and to help your body and mind get back into balance than a good old-fashioned chuckle. Laughing is also a powerful antidote to conflict and stress that helps boost the immune system, relaxes the entire body, releases endorphins, and tones your belly. It can lighten your load, help you connect with others, and keep you grounded. Give yourself the gift of laughter today by watching a romantic comedy or calling an old friend to chat about fond and funny memories. Whatever is sure to give you a hearty laugh, that's what you want to be doing today.

DAY 20

What's Holding You Back?

Back of Core

Now that you've thoroughly worked the front of your core, let's turn our attention to the back of the core for balance and further reduction of the muffin top. But more than that, this part of your body also shows you how you hold back in your body and in your life. Our ultimate goal is for the spine and back of the core to be fluid, flexible, and strong. You want your movement to originate in the core and then move out from there through your entire body. More important, you are learning how to let go and come into your own authentic power.

Today I want you to take a look at those situations in life where it's difficult for you to be up- front, and how holding back causes you to put up a good front. *Where am I holding back in my life? Where am I not expressing myself or not doing the things I want to do? Do I live my life focused on the past? Where am I holding back on making decisions in my life, and how can I begin to move forward?*

Spinal Roll-down

- Stand up tall against a wall with your feet hip width apart, knees soft, your head and tail touching the wall, and your legs and feet slightly away from it.
- Inhale and bend your knees slightly. Then exhale while you slowly peel yourself away from the wall one vertebra at a time until you are hanging forward, your neck and shoulders relaxed.
- Bend your knees another few inches while your tush slides down the wall.
- Extend your knees (still leaving a soft bend in them) as you slowly come back up to stand, sliding your tush and sitz bones back up to release the back of your core and hamstrings.

Repeat this movement six times.

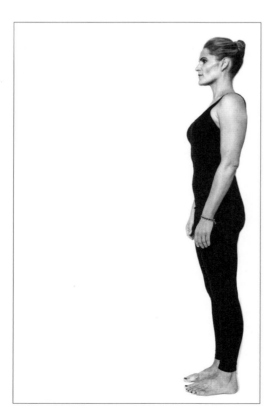
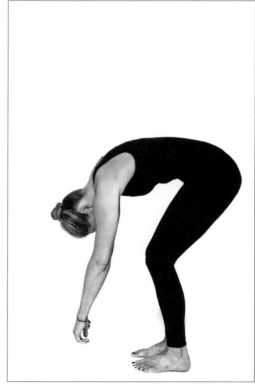

QL Roll

- Place the roller behind you.
- Come to a figure-four position with your left knee bent, right ankle crossed over your left thigh, right above the knee. Your forearms should be on the mat, palms on the roller, thumbs facing in. Lean your body to the right while feeling a subtle pressure on the right quadratus lumborum (QL), a lower back muscle between the bottom of your ribs and the top of your hips.
- Keeping the roller stable, press down into your foot while you inhale and curl your tailbone up; exhale and come back down.

Repeat this movement eight times on each side, alternating sides.

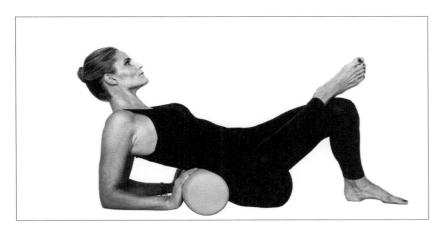

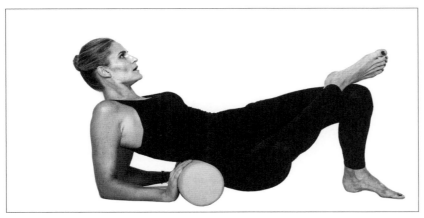

Roll Like a Ball

- Sit on the mat with your knees bent and bring the roller in front of your shins, holding on to either end of it with your hands. Relax your shoulders, broaden your back, deepen your abdominals, and make a balanced C-shaped curve of your spine from head to tail. Lift your feet off the mat and balance on or just behind your sitz bones.

- Inhale as you pull your lower abs in and let gravity roll you back to the top of your shoulders, smoothing out the tissue of your entire spine. Maintain the C-shape.

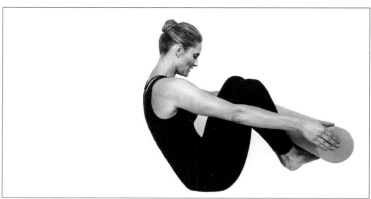

- Exhale as you return to the upright position and pause to balance, all the while keeping your belly scooped and your spine in a C-curve.

Repeat this movement eight times.

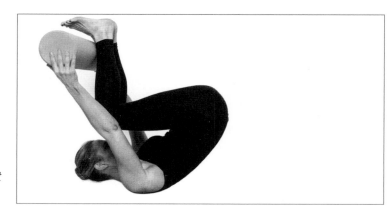

RESHAPE

Roll-up

- Lie down on the mat faceup with the roller underneath the back of your lower calves.
- Inhale as you curl your chin to your chest and round your spine up and over like a cresting wave.
- Exhale as you round all the way forward, soften your knees, and pull your navel to your spine to create a U-shape with your entire body.
- Inhale as you begin to roll your spine down one vertebra at a time. Exhale to finish rolling all the way back down to the mat, scooping your belly and releasing your hips and lower back.

Repeat this movement six to eight times.

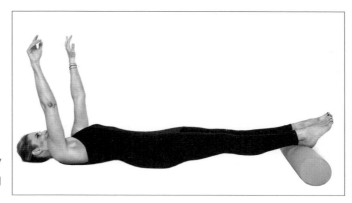

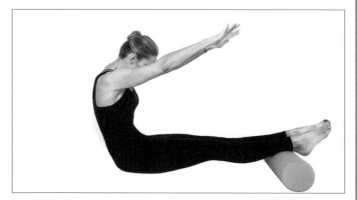

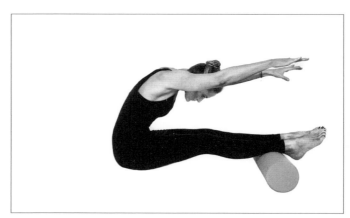

Rollover with Leg Circles

- Lie down on the mat with the roller placed just above your sacrum so that your hips are on the roller, with legs extended toward the ceiling. Place your palms on top of the roller, with your elbows slightly bent to open your shoulders and chest and engage your triceps.
- Inhale to lower your legs down to a 45-degree angle, keeping your core strong to avoid straining your lower back.
- Exhale and start rolling over into an inverted U-shape, keeping your body suspended and abs and hamstrings engaged.
- Inhale as you slowly roll your spine down one vertebra at a time, while also opening your legs out to the side and, with control, lowering them down.
- Exhale as you draw your legs back up to a 45-degree angle. Abs, legs, and triceps should be activated while your spine decompresses.

Repeat this movement six times.

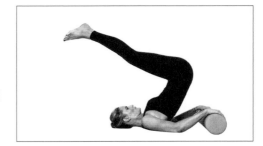

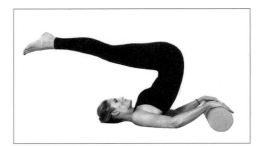

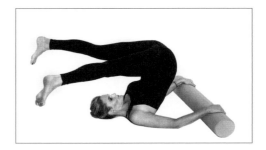

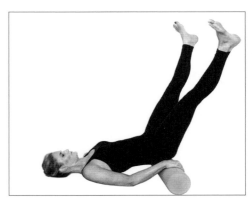

Emotional Benefits

- Enhances self-expression self-knowledge.
- Deepens emotional connection.
- Creates a sense of ease in communicating your emotions.
- Results in a deeper sense of self.
- Tunes you in to your desires.
- Ease in being yourself.

SELF-CARE SECOND

Vision boards are a great way to define what you want and to remind yourself of your goals and desires on a daily basis. They allow you to align yourself with your higher self and authentic purpose, and to create the life you really want. Many consider a vision board to be a vital step along the road to success. Since positive, focused thinking is key to achieving goals, pinpointing what those goals are and having something tangible to symbolize them are essential parts of the process. Vision boards remind you of what you should and should not be doing in order to achieve your goals. The images and phrases on the board should represent the highest priorities in your life. How do you know what you want until you actually define it.

Find pictures that represent or symbolize the experiences, feelings, and things you want to attract into your life, as well as those things that bring meaning and purpose to your life. Take your time choosing photographs, magazine cut-outs, pictures, and postcards—whatever inspires or speaks to you. Be creative and joyful in this process! When you've finished collecting your images, pin them on a corkboard. This board will serve as a means of reinforcing what you truly want in your life and will help keep you on track. Put it somewhere you will see it every day so the images can imprint themselves on your subconscious.

Getting Out of Your Head

Collarbone, Neck, Jaw, and Face

Congratulations on reaching the final day of the program! We're ending with the collarbone, neck, jaw, and face, which seems appropriate because I always like to think of this part of the body as our champagne cork. So let's pop that cork to celebrate reaching the end of this journey—or at least the first chapter of it!

This sequence will restore alignment and tone to your neck, and decrease stress in your head and jaw to help reveal that long and lean ballerina neck. It will also help you return to a more balanced relationship between your mind and body, and between your own mental reasoning and your inner knowing. Physically, the work you do here can dramatically restore and delay the aging process in your head, neck, and face. Releasing excess mental tension and calming the overactive mind is also huge when it comes to fostering and restoring a youthful demeanor.

A few things to ponder as you end your 21-day journey: *Do I like to have rational answers for everything? To what extent do my feelings and thought processes guide me in life? Am I an overthinker? Do I get stuck in my head too much?* Pay attention during those moments when you "go into your head" or when you become too involved in thinking, figuring things out, and trying to make things happen. In those moments, make a concerted effort to relax the muscles in your head, face, jaw, and neck to help you look and *feel* younger and more at peace.

WARM-UP

Neck Twist with Jaw Stretch

- Come to a seated position on your roller and reach your arms behind you. Interlace your fingers and press your knuckles down toward the mat behind you.
- Keeping your chest open and lifted, inhale as you turn your head to the right. Exhale completely; then lift your chin up and extend your lower jaw away from your neck, creating an underbite with your jaw. Relax the jaw and inhale to return to center.

Repeat this movement six to eight times per side, alternating sides.

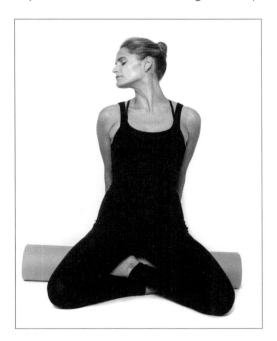

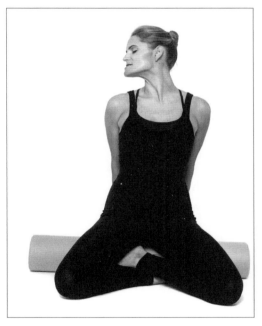

Collarbone Alignment

- Place the roller behind your upper back with your elbows bent and palms up. Bend your knees and plant your feet on the floor together.
- Exhale as you simultaneously lower your knees to the left and look to the right.
- Inhale to lift back to center and then exhale as you lower your knees to the right and look to the left. Inhale to lift back to center.

Repeat this movement eight times to each side.

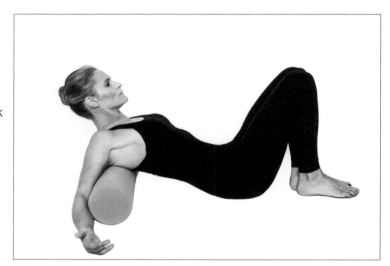

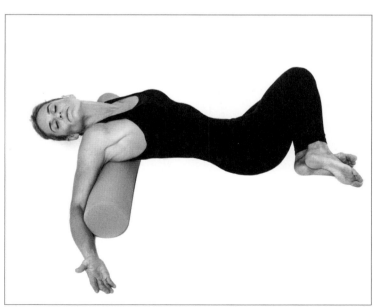

Neck Massage

- Lie down on your back and place the roller at the base of your skull, putting your hands on either end to stretch the arms and keep it steady.
- Inhale and turn your head to the left, feeling the roller gently massage your neck.
- Exhale as you return back to center.
- Inhale to fully rotate your neck to the right. Exhale to return to center.

Repeat this movement eight times on each side.

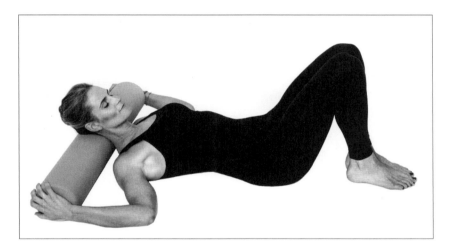

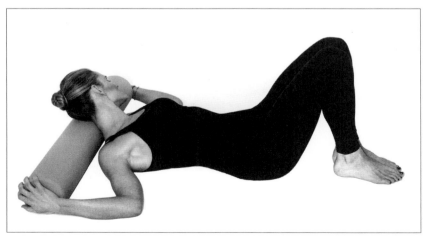

Rolling Mermaid Twist with Neck Stretch

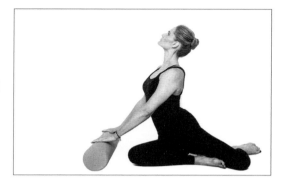

- Place your right shin in front of you and your left shin out to the left side so that your knees are staggered. Place the roller to the right of you and put the palm of your right hand on the roller. Pull up and lift your sides and lift through the top of your head.

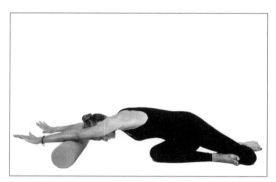

- Inhaling, roll the roller up your forearms to just below your elbows.
- Exhale as you roll back up to the starting position.
- Inhale as you windmill your arms up and over to the left, placing your left hand on the floor slightly behind your left knee and wrapping your right hand around your left ear.

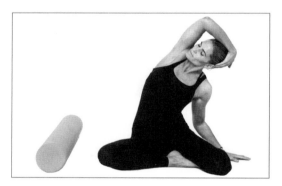

- Exhale as you curl and twist, drawing your right elbow toward your left knee to round down and open up the right side of your neck.
- Inhale to lift back up to center.

Repeat this motion six to eight times, then repeat on the other side.

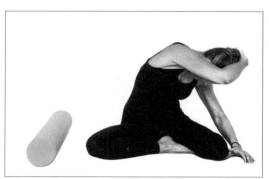

RESHAPE

Rolling Swan with Neck Twist

• Lie belly-down on the mat, with arms long in front of you and the roller placed just below your elbow joints, thumbs facing up. Reach your heels away from your heart to feel oppositional energy and decompress your spine.

• Inhale and roll the roller toward you, extending your spine and lifting your heart as you roll your shoulders back (taking care to keep your glutes relaxed the entire time so you don't jam your lower back while lifting up). Exhale to come all the way up to the top, being sure to pull your abs up and in.

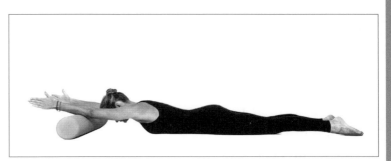

• While you are holding yourself up in extension, inhale and turn your head to the right. Exhale to return to center. Then turn to the left as you inhale. Exhale to return to center once again.

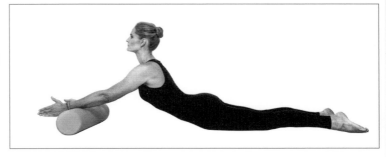

• Inhale as you begin to lower down, slowly resisting as you go; exhale as you come all the way down.

Repeat this movement eight times.

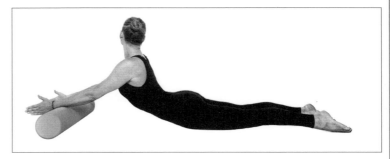

Emotional Benefits

- Gets you out of your head and enjoying the present.
- Creates a connection to your inner knowing/third eye.
- Reduces overthinking.
- Helps keep you from trying so hard.

SELF-CARE SECOND

A self scalp massage can be incredibly therapeutic. The tension will literally melt away not only from your head but also from your entire body. It can even help improve sleep, de-stress your mind, relax your nervous system, and stimulate hair growth. It's a simple and effective technique that you can do anywhere at any time.

Start by using your index and middle fingers to gently massage small circles on your temples. Gradually move your fingers over the rest of your scalp, maintaining an even, enjoyable pressure as you work from the hairline back to the base of the skull. This pressure on the sensitive and receptive scalp area will help calm the body and mind and release all of the tension we store from the overstimulation of daily life.

You've now completed the first round of my total body "recipe". Fantastic work! Take a moment to honor the fact that you have learned some amazing new ways to enhance your shape and presence and that you have committed to making them a daily ritual. You are on your way to a longer, leaner, calmer and more youthful you. Bravo!

Now keep things rolling ... move on to exercises to align your body with your mind!

Roller Rx

While the 21-day program will give you the jump-start you need to get your body and mind humming along in tandem like a well-oiled machine, the truth is that life still happens. Many of us deal with chronic issues or have physical and emotional reactions to particularly stressful or rocky times that require a little bit of extra maintenance or TLC for specific aspects of our well-being.

The rolling exercises that follow are designed to give you that extra spot treatment and pick-me-up as you need it, whether it's for a bout of insomnia or a spurt of anxiety. Whenever you need a little bit of Rx, just flip through these pages to find the series of movements that will best relax your body and soothe your soul in the moment at hand.

Rolling for Anxiety

Feelings of worry, fear, and tension are a totally normal reaction to stress; however, a constant state of anxiety or excessive levels of it may be symptomatic of an anxiety disorder. Anxiety disorders—or experiencing fear, worry, panic, or anxiety in common or normal situations—are the most common disruption in brain health in the United States. In fact, according to the National Institue of Mental Health, it affects 40 million adults, about 18% of the population. Physical signs that you may have an anxiety disorder include sudden panic attacks without any real trigger, headaches, fatigue, tension, difficulty swallowing, trembling, twitching, irritability, sweating, and hot flashes. Emotional symptoms include worry, fear, overthinking, and feelings of doom.

Those who are plagued with anxiety may live with a constant nagging worry or overall anxiousness that can restrict their ability to maintain relationships, work, or even leave the house. Anxiety activates our fight-or-flight mechanism, even when there aren't any real risks or threats. The fear of being in danger never goes away. The good news is that incorporating mind-body movements into your regular routine is one of the best ways to clear your head and rejuvenate your spirit.

Think of this sequence as a mental nap that will tune you in to your body and slow down the monkey-mind chatter in your head by allowing you to focus on deep breathing and the moment at hand. The following movements will help you become more grounded and calmer, soothe your nervous system, and melt away tension. Restorative poses, inversions, and forward bends are especially calming to the body and mind, helping to reduce and prevent excessive anxiety. Back-bends strengthen the legs, open the chest, and stimulate the abdominal organs, lungs, and thyroid, which reduces anxiety, calms the central nervous system, and relaxes the mind, while strengthening the spine, hips, and neck. Time to open up and roll away your mental stress!

Roll Out the Kinks (page 99)
Roll-up (page 161)
Bridge (page 51)
Standing Chest Expansion (page 22)

Bid Your Anxiety Adieu

• **Warm yourself up.** Research has found that heating up your body reduces tension and anxiety. Warm sensations like the sun on your back, a warm bath, a sauna, a cozy lit fireplace, or a cup of warm tea may alter neurotransmitters that control mood, including serotonin. Add some lavender essential oil to your bath for a relaxing and calming effect.

• **Eat your eggs.** Eggs are one of nature's best sources of B vitamins, which are crucial for brain health.

• **Indulge in a bit of chocolate!** Here's some good news: Mood-enhancing organic dark chocolate without added sugars or dairy is a great option for alleviating anxiety. It's known to reduce cortisol, the stress hormone that causes anxiety.

• **Make a gratitude list.** Studies have shown that expressing gratitude can help reduce anxiety. Get into the glass-half-full mindset and start a gratitude journal to help you feel less overwhelmed.

• **At-home acupressure.** Press the webbing between your thumb and index finger. Bringing circulation to this point helps reduce muscle tension, stress, and anxiety.

Rolling the Blues Away

Depression affects more than 350 million people worldwide. It is a disempowering condition that can influence your family life, work, and school, and can even disrupt eating, sleeping, and general health habits. Unfortunately, in the United States, depression has increased dramatically every year over the course of the past century. Depression usually presents itself as low energy, a sad mood, low self-esteem, a loss of interest, and a loss of pleasure, and can include emotions of anger, hopelessness, and despair. Typically, depressed people have lower levels of energy; it's harder for them to deal with daily stresses, and they often feel overwhelmed by normal daily tasks and relationships. We ladies have to be particularly on guard because women are 70 percent more likely than men to experience depression in their lifetime.

This sequence includes restorative moves, fear-conquering backbends, and a means for the mind to release heavy thoughts and the body to let go of tension.

Standing Chest Expansion (page 22)
Arm Circles (page 98)
Psoas Backbend Twist (page 74)

Bring Some Light into Your Life

• **Get your vitamin D on.** Most people in the United States are deficient in vitamin D, also known as the sunshine vitamin. A sunny day will always boost your mood, and now studies show that it may even increase levels of the mood-lifting chemical serotonin. To get your daily dose of D, spend twenty minutes outside sans sunscreen or take a vitamin D sublingual supplement.
• **Treat yourself to some acupuncture.** Studies show that acupuncture is a great

option for treating depression. When the needle goes in, your body responds by releasing endorphins, which help you feel happy, calm, relaxed, and less defeated.

- **Snack on some pumpkin seeds.** Pumpkin seeds are a great way to combat the blues, since they contain magnesium, tryptophan, and omega-3 fats, which help nourish the brain, lighten your mood, and boost the production of serotonin.

Rolling for Digestion and to Banish Bloating

Efficient digestion is the key to radiant health. Bloating, constipation, irritable bowel syndrome (IBS), and belly discomfort and pain are all signs of a sluggish or stressed digestive tract. Enhancing digestion leads to regular elimination, which is the body's way of flushing toxins and staying vibrant. When digestion is slow and imbalanced, disease thrives. Even the common cold comes from an energy imbalance that begins in the digestive tract.

Luckily, rolling offers an amazing tool for improving digestive function by helping the body move food through the intestines and improving circulation to the belly area. It can even reduce inflammation. Plus, by decreasing stress and calming the sympathetic nervous system, rolling can help regulate and enhance digestion. The twisting moves included in this sequence apply gentle pressure to the belly, like an internal massage for your intestines.

Of course, the food we eat also plays a big role in how efficiently we digest it. This sequence will give you a deeper awareness of your belly and its needs. Because of this, after a while, you will find yourself making better food choices, craving less sugar, and choosing foods that truly give you life force (or *chi*) and bring a deeper sense of balance, harmony, and well-being.

This sequence of forward folds and twists supported by deep breaths will help stimulate the abdominal organs while also increasing the efficiency of the bowels, thus relieving constipation and helping to minimize belching and gas.

Snow Angels (page 23)
Roller Saw (page 196)
Roll-up (page 161)
Rolling Swan (page 26)

Banish Bloat

- **Drink probiotics.** Probiotics are the "good" gut bacteria. Studies show that they can help alleviate digestive problems and boost immunity. These natural microbes can be found as supplements and in cultured foods and yogurts. I love to add organic plain whole milk Lifeway kefir with no added sugars or flavors to my morning smoothie. You can find Lifeway kefir at laurenroxburgh.com.
- **Sip ginger tea.** The anti-inflammatory and antibacterial properties in ginger can relax the belly, calm digestive spasms, and relieve gas, nausea, indigestion, and even bloating. Chop and peel a few slices of ginger and simmer them in boiling water to make ginger tea.
- **Chew fennel seeds or sip fennel tea.** Fennel (which tastes like a mild licorice) does an amazing job of relaxing the colon. This remedy has been used in Ayurvedic and European medical practices for centuries. Snacking on fennel seeds or sipping them in your tea will prevent and treat bloating, constipation, and gas. It also helps promote the secretion of digestive enzymes that lower appetite in a healthy way and aids in the release of excess water weight. In India, these seeds are routinely chewed after meals to promote digestion.
- **Rebound.** Here's yet another reason rebounding is your greatest ally! Rebounding for a few minutes a day enhances digestion and elimination. Just wait a few hours after eating to avoid bouncing on a full tummy. My favorite rebounder is Bellicon, which you can find at laurenroxburgh.com.

Rolling for Insomnia

Insomnia is one of the most common issues in the United States, affecting over half of all Americans. Insomnia is the inability to fall asleep or remain asleep long enough to feel rested and rejuvenated, especially when the problem continues over time. The world looks so much more stressful and overwhelming when you're not rested. But don't fret—there *is* relief! The following routine will help you connect with your body and breath to help release tension and calm your mind. This combination of movement and breath regulates your nervous system to reduce stress and help you be present and sleep better. Just follow this pre-bedtime time routine to help take the "weight of the world" off your shoulders and melt your way to a peaceful slumber.

Roll Out the Kinks (page 99)
Snow Angels (page 23)
Rolling Mermaid Twist (page 90)

Preparing for Mr. Sandman

- **Make your bedroom a technology-free zone.** The artificial blue light emitted by illuminated devices activates the brain and makes it harder to sleep.
- **Meditate.** Play your day backward in your mind and feel yourself slip away to slumberland.
- **Pop some magnesium.** It's the most powerful mineral for relaxation available, and science says it can dramatically improve sleep. Take 400 to 500 milligrams before you go to sleep. I like Natural Calm, the only water-soluble magnesium blend.
- **Take a hot soak in a magnesium chloride bath.** Incorporating this ritual into your pre-bedtime routine will calm your body's nervous system, naturally relax your muscles, and help you get some deep, quality z's.
- **Make your bed.** According to the National Sleep Foundation, it turns out that people who make their bed regularly are 19 percent more likely to sleep.

Rolling for Migraines and Headaches

Headaches (and migraines, especially) have a special way of completely disrupting a person's life. According to the Migraine Research Foundation, migraines affect more than 36 million people in the United States, most often females. Hormones, stress, tension, dehydration, and diet can all be triggers.

A regular restorative roller routine that incorporates mindful breathing and relaxation can help prevent or reduce the severity of headaches and migraines. If you practice these roller moves, your self-awareness will increase and help guide you to the source of your pain. These moves will dramatically improve circulation, promote the flow of oxygenated blood directly to the brain, decrease stress, and reduce pain. Serotonin levels decrease when you're in the throes of a migraine, but the good news is that these specific moves will help give them a boost! Focus on slow, rhythmic breathing to help calm your nervous system and relax your body and mind.

Spinal Roll-down (page 58)
Slinky Spine (page 80)
Rolling Mermaid Twist (page 90)
Inverted Sacral Roll (page 194)

Say Hello to a Healthier Head

- **Take a power nap.** A simple twenty-minute nap is enough for your body to reboot. It will release stress, regulate your systems, and relieve your head. Be sure not to rest for longer than twenty minutes so as not to affect your regular sleep cycle.
- **Get pepperminty.** Peppermint has been used as an anti-inflammatory remedy in both Chinese medicine and old-school European herbal medicine for centuries. You can massage it into your temples as an essential oil or sip on some peppermint tea.
- **Pop some magnesium.** Studies have shown a link to a magnesium deficiency and migraines. This mineral can help relax the body's muscle and nerve impulses. My favorite is Calm.

All Rolled Into One

A Glossary of Foam Roller Exercises

by Body Part

Here you'll find in-depth descriptions of every sequence contained within this book. Feel free to flip to specific exercises as you go through each of the twenty-one days of the program or the Roller Rx series to find each movement outlined on a step-by-step basis. You can also use this section to put together your own rolling program for targeted movement exercises.

I have divided all of the exercises in this book into specific areas of the body. If you feel like your thighs need a little extra love, flip to the section of this chapter covering thigh work either to add a few extra movements into your 21-day rolling routine or for a stand-alone targeted thigh workout. Feel like powering up your core? Just flip to that section to add a little fire to your belly.

Feel free to experiment, mix it up, and give your body what it needs with this comprehensive movement section.

ARMS

Reverse Push-Through

- Place the roller horizontally about a foot behind you. Sit up tall with your legs long out in front of you. Reach behind you to place your palms facedown on the roller, thumbs pointing out.

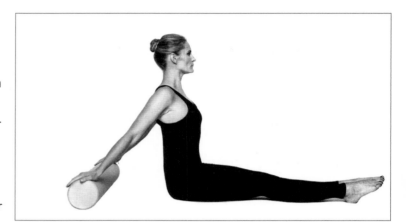

- Inhale as you scoop your tail under, placing some weight onto the roller. As you roll back, scoop your belly as the roller rolls up your wrists and forearms to just below your elbow joints. You will end up with a long spine and your arms, shoulders, and chest stretched open.

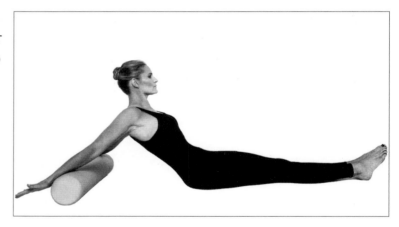

- Exhale as you slowly roll back up to a tall spine, sitting on your sitz bones.

Repeat this movement six times.

Reverse Triceps Dip

- Sit down on the mat and place the roller behind you. Place your palms firmly down on the roller shoulder-width apart, with your pinkie fingers facing out. Press your feet into the mat to lift your tush off the floor. Open your chest, lengthen your neck, and draw your shoulders back.

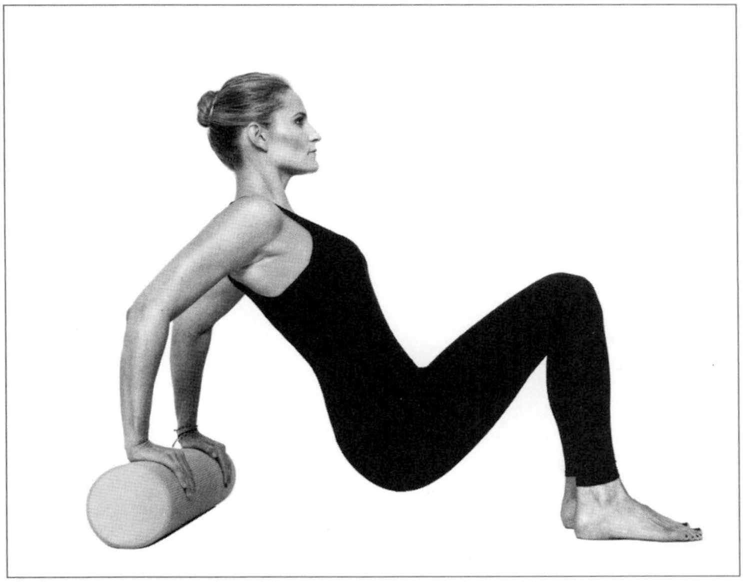

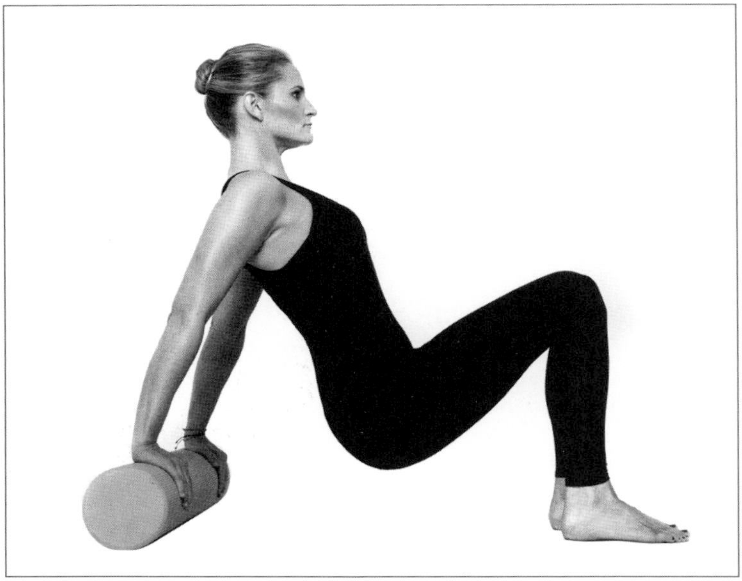

- Bend your knees up toward the ceiling so that your heels are directly under your knees. Plant your feet firmly on the floor hip width apart, lift your hips up, and straighten your arms.
- Keeping the roller stable, your core engaged, and your chest open to avoid hunching, inhale as you slowly bend your elbows behind you.
- Exhale as you press up to a soft elbow, taking care to avoid locking the elbow joints.

Repeat this movement ten times.

Rolling Swan

- Lie belly-down on the mat, with arms long in front of you and the roller placed just below your elbow joints, thumbs facing up. Reach your heels away from your heart to feel oppositional energy and decompress your spine.
- Inhale and roll the roller toward you, extending your spine and lifting your heart as you roll your shoulders back (taking care to keep your glutes relaxed the entire time so you don't jam your lower back while lifting up). Be sure to pull your abs up and in to support your back and elongate the front of your body.
- Exhale as you slowly resist on the way down, returning to the position you started in.

Repeat this movement eight times.

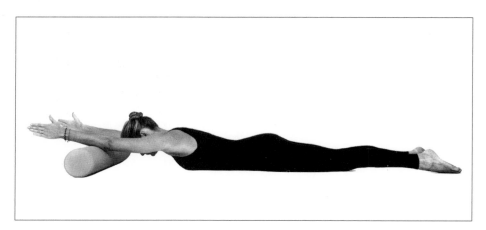

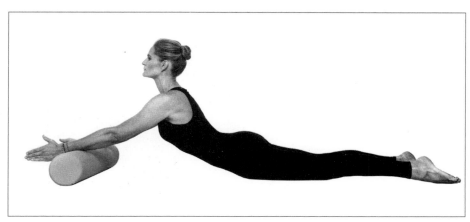

Rolling Swan with Arm Pulls

- Lie belly-down on the mat, with arms long in front of you and the roller placed just below your elbow joints, thumbs facing up. Reach your heels away from your heart to feel oppositional energy and decompress your spine.
- Inhale and roll the roller toward you, extending your spine and lifting your heart as you roll your shoulders back (taking care to keep your glutes relaxed the entire time so you don't jam your lower back while lifting up). Be sure to pull your abs in and up to support your back and elongate the front of your body.

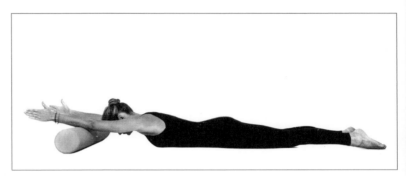

- Remaining in this suspended position and keeping your shoulders drawn down, exhale as you pull your elbows back toward you. Continue to remain suspended as you inhale to straighten your arms. Repeat this arm pull six times.

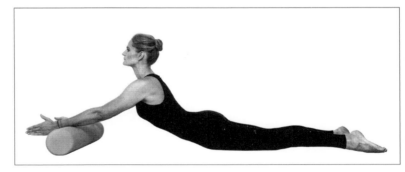

- Exhale again as you slowly resist on the way down, returning to the starting position.

Repeat this movement eight times.

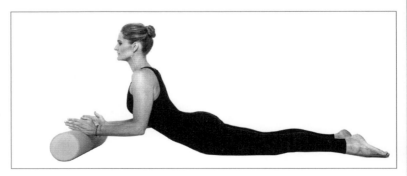

Rollover with Arm Presses

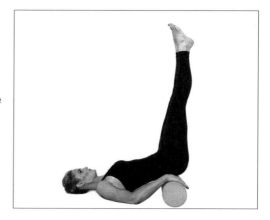

- Lie down on the mat with the roller placed just above your sacrum so that your hips are on the roller, with legs extended toward the ceiling. Place your palms on top of the roller, with your elbows slightly bent to open your shoulders and chest and engage your triceps.
- Inhale to lower your legs down to a 45-degree angle, keeping your core strong to avoid loading your lower back.
- Exhale and start rolling over into an inverted U-shape, keeping your body suspended and abs and hamstrings engaged.
- Inhale again as you slowly roll your body halfway down, decompressing your spine and activating your triceps.
- Exhale as you return to the starting position.

Repeat this movement six times.

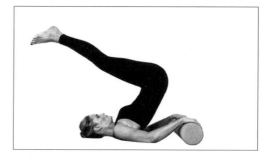

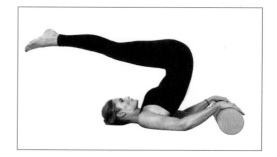

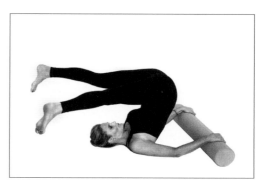

CHEST

Diaphragm Release

- Place the roller underneath the bottom of your shoulder blades (at the bra line, for the ladies). Gently interlace your fingers and bring your hands behind your head to support your neck. Place your feet on the floor, with knees bent and feet hip width apart.
- Inhale as you arch your thoracic spine (or middle to upper back) over the roller.
- Exhale as you curl back up as if you were doing a crunch, squeezing all the air out of your stomach.

Repeat this movement eight to ten times.

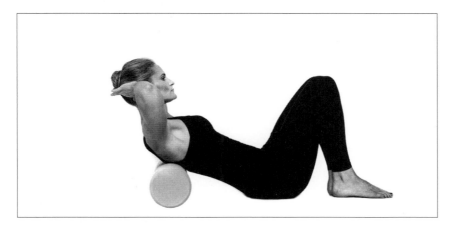

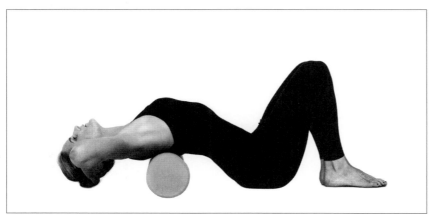

Diaphragm Release with Organ Twist

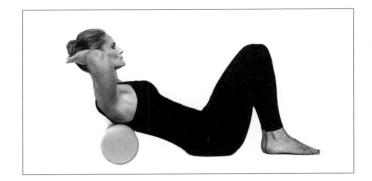

- Lie on the mat with the roller placed under your back at the bra line. Gently interlace your fingers behind your head to support your head and neck.
- Inhale as you arch your thoracic spine (or middle to upper back) over the roller.
- Exhale as you twist your legs and hips to the left, squeezing and wringing out your organs.
- Inhale to bring your knees to center and repeat this motion on the other side.

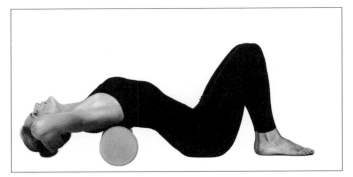

Repeat this movement eight to ten times on each side, alternating sides.

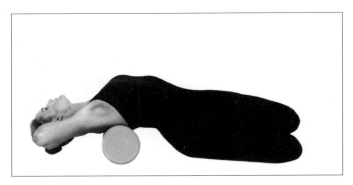

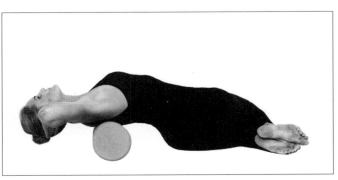

Standing Chest Expansion

- Come to a standing position with your feet hip width apart and a soft knees. Hold your arms out to the side with a slight bend in the elbows, palms facing forward and fingers pointing up.
- Inhale as you reach your right arm behind you and twist your body to the right to expand your chest, lungs, and arms.
- Exhale as you come back through center and reach your left arm behind you as you twist to the left.

Repeat this movement ten times.

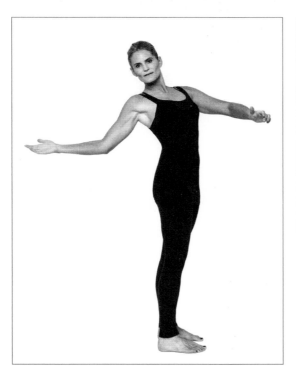 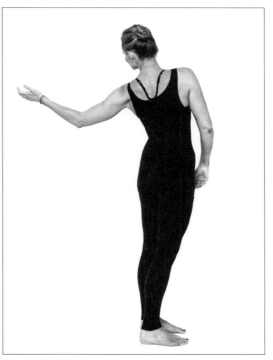

90-Degree Psoas Roll

• Come down to your forearms with the roller placed perpendicular under your left hip. Bend your left knee so that your heel is pointing toward the ceiling. Place your right inner knee and thigh parallel to the roller.

• Twist your body slightly to the right to expose your psoas, and roll up and down the attachment of your hip and psoas, keeping your breath smooth as you move. (Note that this is a very small and slow movement—you'll be rolling no more than two inches.)

Repeat this movement eight times, then repeat on the other side.

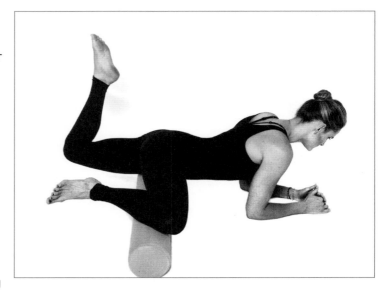

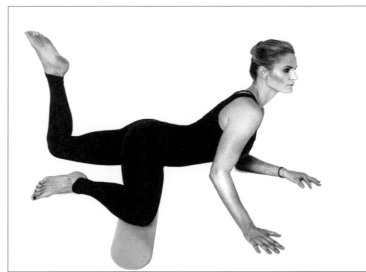

Balancing Core Work

- Lie on the roller with a neutral spine, with the roller supporting you from head to tailbone. Place your forearms on either side of the roller to stabilize. Lift your legs with your knees bent at a 90-degree angle, with your heels together and toes apart. Your knees should be shoulder-width apart.
- Lift your shoulder blades off the roller and curl up over your bra line, keeping a long neck.
- Keeping your curl engaged, inhale and extend your legs out to no lower than a 45-degree angle.
- Exhale as you bend knees back in while you maintain your curl.

Repeat this movement eight to ten times on each side, alternating sides.

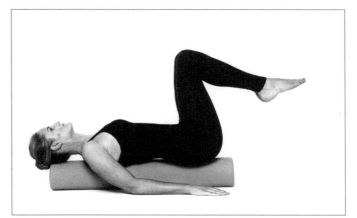

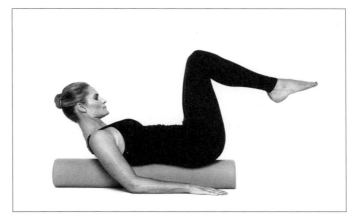

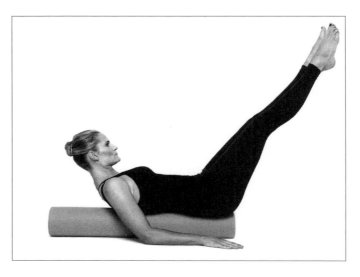

Grasshopper

- Place your lower thighs (right above your kneecaps) on the roller and your hands directly under your shoulders, fingers pointing forward. Inhale to bring your spine into extension, looking straight ahead.
- Exhale and bend your elbows to lower down, hovering over the mat.
- Inhale and return to your starting position.

Repeat this movement eight to ten times.

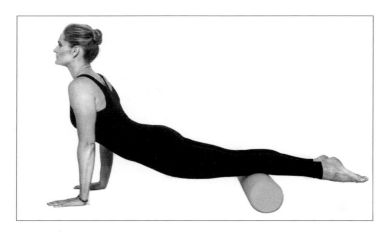

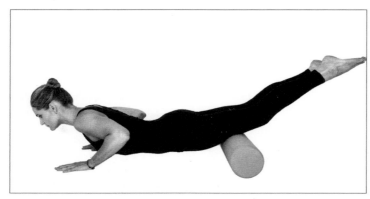

Inverted Core Series

- Lie down on the mat and place the roller under your sacrum. Keeping your upper back and shoulders on the mat, elevate your waist to a bridge position while maintaining a neutral spine. Bring your knees over your hips and then extend your legs to about a 90-degree angle so they're pointing up to the ceiling. Place your hands on either side of the outer edge of the roller to keep it stable throughout the exercise. Note that your spine should remain stable and neutral for the duration of this exercise.

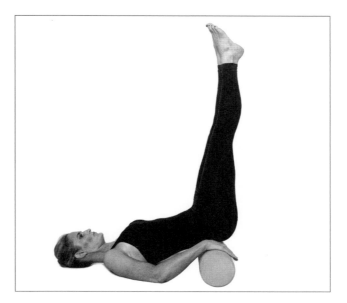

- Inhale as you slowly lower your legs down toward your mat. Bring them down as low as you can without any sensation or arching in your lower back or shoulders.

- Exhale as you use your deep lower belly to draw your legs back up toward the ceiling to 90 degrees.

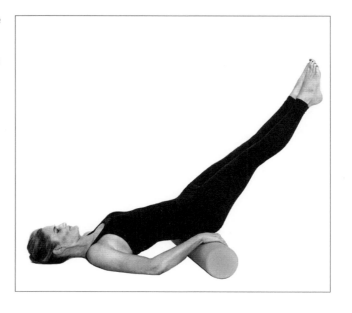

Repeat this movement eight to ten times.

Inverted Sacral Roll

- Place the roller under your sacrum (the triangular bone at the base of your spine).
- Place your upper back and shoulders on the mat, keeping your waist elevated in a bridge position. Lift your legs to a 90-degree angle so they're pointing up to the ceiling.
- Place your hands on either side of the outer edge of the roller to make sure it doesn't slip. The roller will remain stable throughout this exercise.
- Inhale as you begin lowering your legs down toward your face. Bring them down as low as you can without sensation or arching in your lower back and/or shoulders.
- As you exhale, use your deep lower belly to draw your legs back up toward the ceiling. Your spine should remain stable and neutral for the duration of this exercise.

Repeat this movement eight to ten times.

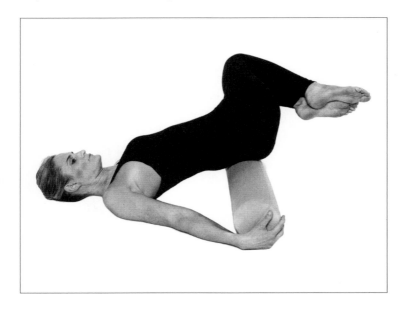

Psoas Rolling Lunge Twist

- Stand on your right foot with your right knee slightly bent, and put the top of your left foot on the roller behind you with your back leg straight. Raise your arms directly overhead.
- Inhale as you bend your right knee, keeping the knee over the heel, and extend your left hip and leg back, pressing into the foam roller as it rolls up your shin until your right thigh is nearly parallel to the floor.
- Exhale as you twist your body and arms to the right to stretch the psoas.
- Inhale to unwind back to center, and exhale to return to the starting position.

Repeat this movement eight times, then repeat on the other side.

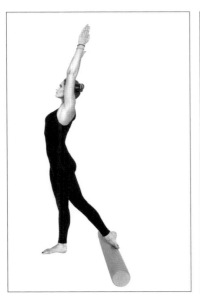 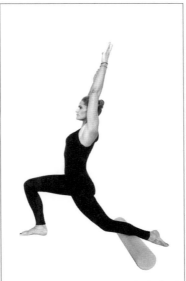 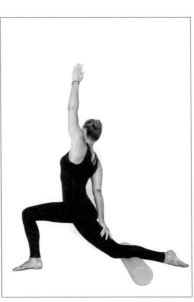

Roller Saw

- Bring your sitz bones to the roller and sit up tall, extending your legs long in front of you and slightly wider than your hips. Reach your arms out to the side in a T-shape to activate your lats.
- Inhale as you lift your belly while keeping your shoulders down, and twist your spine to the left.
- Exhale as you reach your right pinkie finger down to "saw" off your left pinkie toe, while keeping your right sitz bone heavy on the roller.
- Inhale as you lift your torso up, still keeping it twisted to the left.
- Exhale as you twist back to center.

Repeat this movement eight times on each side, alternating sides.

Rolling Shell

- Bring the roller right below your knee joint, legs together and extended, toes pointed. Place your hands on the mat shoulder-width apart and stack your shoulders directly above your wrists. Stabilize your shoulders by imagining there is a skewer through your shoulder joints to keep you from rocking back and forth.
- Inhale and start rolling the roller toward you while lifting your core and rounding your spine into flexion; take a full exhale to pull the roller all the way in while your hips lift, scooping your belly and sucking your tummy in.
- Inhale as you resist while slowly lowering back down; exhale to come all the way back to the starting position.

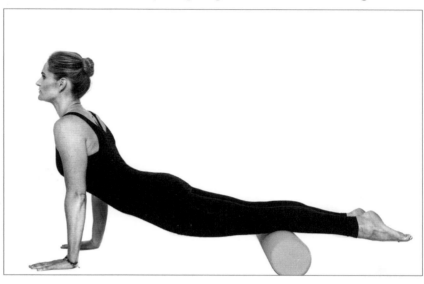

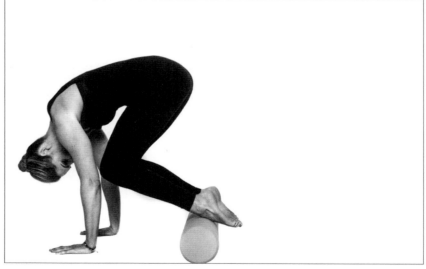

Repeat this movement eight to ten times.

Roll Like a Ball

- Sit on the mat with your knees bent and bring the roller in front of your shins, holding on to either end of it with your hands. Relax your shoulders, broaden your back, deepen your abdominals, and make a balanced C-shaped curve of your spine from head to tail. Lift your feet off the mat and balance on or just behind your sitz bones.

- Inhale as you pull your lower abs in and let gravity roll you back to the top of your shoulders, smoothing out the tissue of your entire spine. Maintain the C-shape.

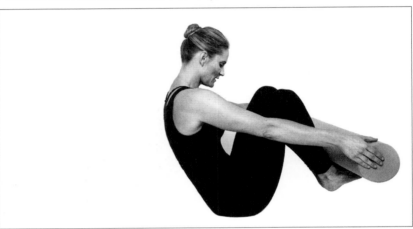

- Exhale as you return to the upright position and pause to balance, all the while keeping your belly scooped and your spine in a C-curve.

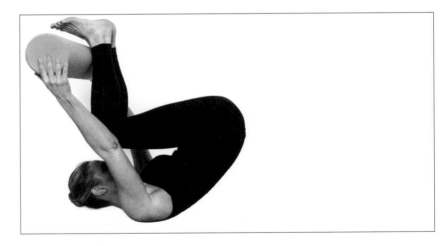

Repeat this movement eight times.

Rollover with Leg Circles

• Lie down on the mat with the roller placed just above your sacrum so that your hips are on the roller, with legs extended toward the ceiling. Place your palms on top of the roller, with your elbows slightly bent to open your shoulders and chest and engage your triceps.

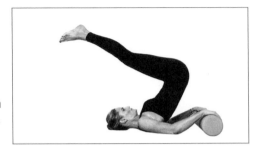

• Inhale to lower your legs down to a 45-degree angle, keeping your core strong to avoid straining your lower back.

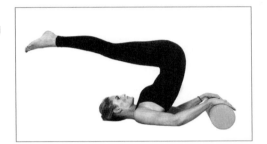

• Exhale and start rolling over into an inverted U-shape, keeping your body suspended and abs and hamstrings engaged.

• Inhale as you slowly roll your spine down one vertebra at a time, while also opening your legs out to the side and, with control, lowering them down.

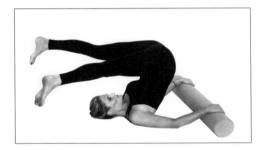

• Exhale as you draw your legs back up to a 45-degree angle. Abs, legs, and triceps should be activated while your spine decompresses.

Repeat this movement six times.

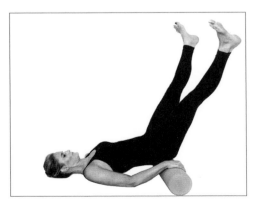

Roll-up

- Lie down on the mat faceup with the roller underneath the back of your lower calves.
- Inhale as you curl your chin to your chest and round your spine up and over like a cresting wave.
- Exhale as you round all the way forward, soften your knees, and pull your navel to your spine to create a U-shape with your entire body.
- Inhale as you begin to roll your spine down one vertebra at a time. Exhale to finish rolling all the way back down to the mat, scooping your belly and releasing your hips and lower back.

Repeat this movement six to eight times.

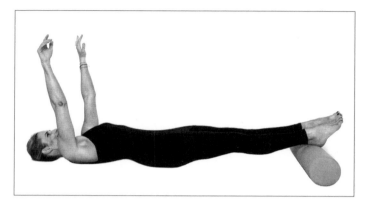

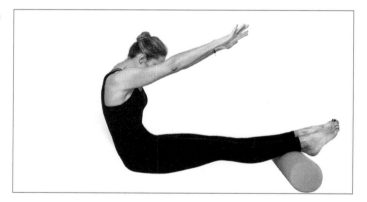

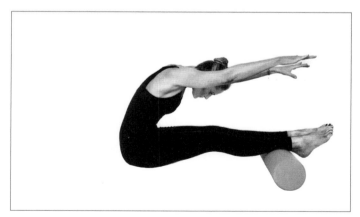

Spinal Roll-down

- Stand up tall against a wall with your feet hip width apart, knees soft, your head and tail touching the wall and your legs and feet slightly away from it.
- Inhale and bend your knees slightly. Then exhale while you slowly peel yourself away from the wall one vertebra at a time until you are hanging forward, your neck and shoulders relaxed.
- Bend your knees another few inches while your tush slides down the wall.
- Extend your knees (still leaving a soft bend in them) as you slowly come back up to stand, sliding your tush and sitz bones back up to release the back of your core and hamstrings.

Repeat this movement six times.

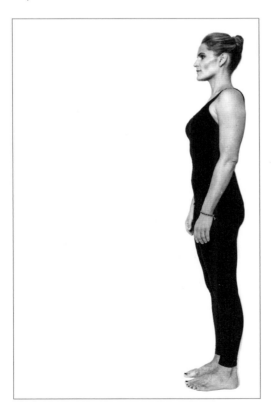 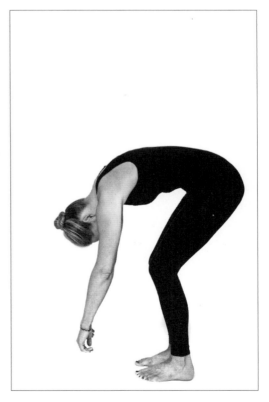

FACE AND NECK

Arms—Back Neck Rolls

- Come to a seated position on your roller and reach your arms behind you. Interlace your fingers and press your knuckles down toward the mat behind you.
- Inhale as you roll your head to the right; exhale as you roll it to the left.
- Next, imagine you have a pencil on your nose and are going to draw a circle. Take your head around in a full circular movement that lasts for an entire inhalation and exhalation. Repeat this movement in the reverse direction.

Repeat each movement eight times on each side and in each direction.

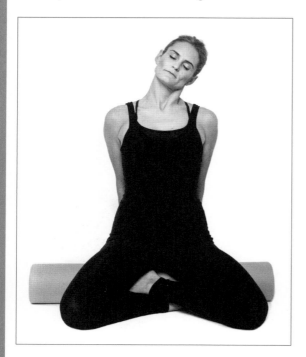 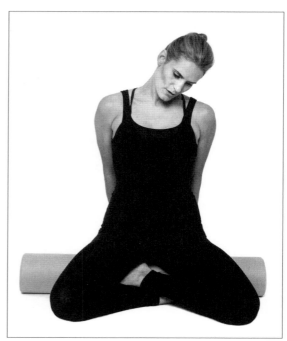

Collarbone Alignment

- Place the roller behind your upper back with your elbows bent and palms up. Bend your knees and plant your feet on the floor together.
- Exhale as you simultaneously lower your knees to the left and look to the right. Inhale to lift back to center and then exhale as you lower your knees to the right and look to the left. Inhale to lift back to center.

Repeat this movement eight times to each side.

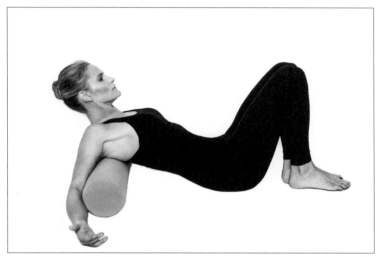

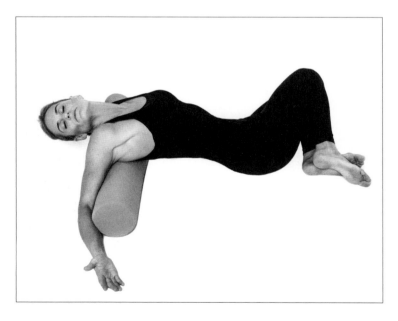

Neck Massage

- Lie down on your back and place the roller at the base of your skull, putting your hands on either end to stretch the arms and keep it steady.
- Inhale and turn your head to the left, feeling the roller gently massage your neck.
- Exhale as you return to center.
- Inhale to fully rotate your neck to the right. Exhale as you return to center

Repeat this movement eight times on each side.

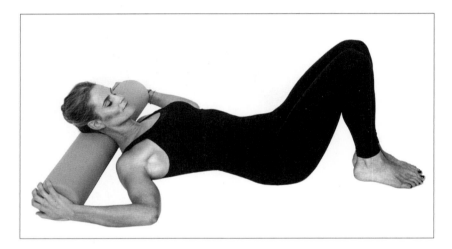

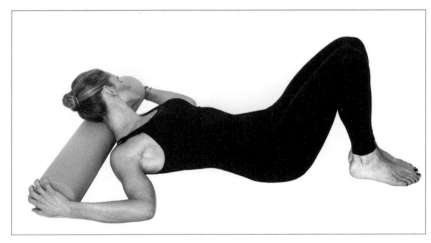

Neck Twist with Jaw Stretch

- Come to a seated position on your roller and reach your arms behind you. Interlace your fingers and press your knuckles down toward the mat behind you.
- Keeping your chest open and lifted, inhale as you turn your head to the right. Exhale completely; then lift your chin up and extend your lower jaw away from your neck, creating an underbite with your jaw. Relax the jaw and inhale to return to center.

Repeat this movement six to eight times per side, alternating sides.

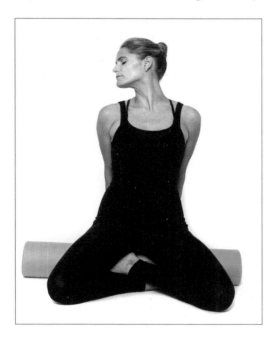 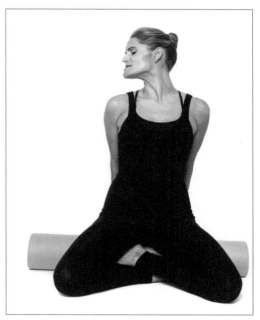

Rolling Mermaid Twist

- Place your right shin in front of you and your left shin out to the left side so that your knees are staggered. Place the roller to the right of you and put the palms of your hands on the roller. Reach and lift your sides and lift through the top of your head.
- Inhale and roll the roller up your forearms to just below your elbows.
- Exhale as you roll back up to the starting position.

Repeat this movement five times, then repeat on the other side.

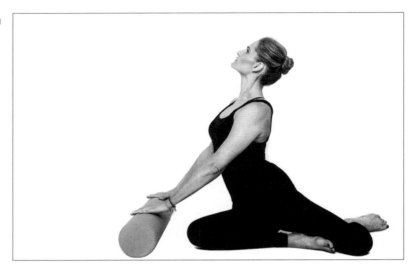

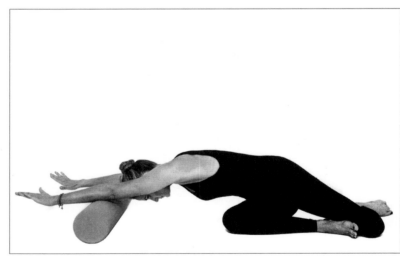

Rolling Mermaid Twist with Neck Stretch

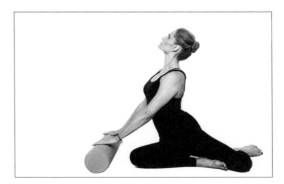

- Place your right shin in front of you and your left shin out to the left side so that your knees are staggered. Place the roller to the right of you and put the palm of your right hand on the roller. Pull up and lift your sides and lift through the top of your head.

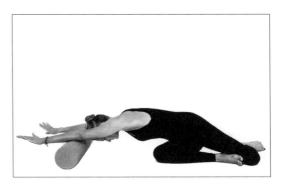

- Inhaling, roll the roller up your forearms to just below your elbows.
- Exhale as you roll back up to the starting position.
- Inhale as you windmill your arms up and over to the left, placing your left hand on the floor slightly behind your left knee and wrapping your right hand around your left ear.

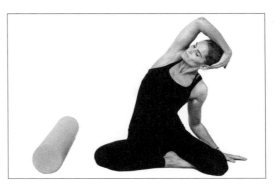

- Exhale as you curl and twist, drawing your right elbow toward your left knee to round down and open up the right side of your neck.
- Inhale to lift back up to center.

Repeat this movement six to eight times, then repeat on the other side.

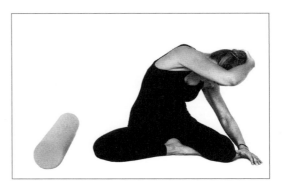

GLUTES

Advanced Grasshopper

- Place your lower thighs (right above your kneecaps) on the roller and your hands directly under your shoulders, fingers pointing forward. Inhale to bring your spine into extension, looking straight ahead.
- Exhale and bend your elbows to lower down, hovering over the mat.
- While hovering, inhale and bend your knees, bringing your heels toward your tush.
- Exhale and extend your legs.
- Inhale and straighten your arms and lift back up; exhale and hold before beginning the next rep.

Repeat this movement eight to ten times.

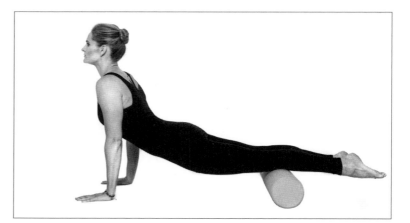

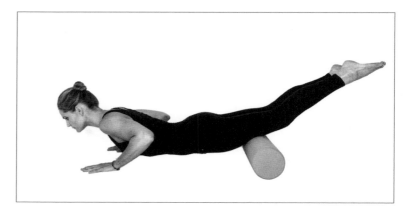

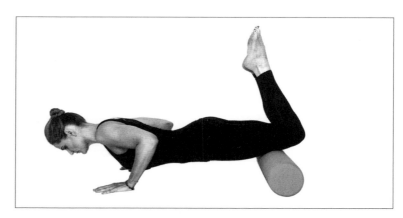

Bridge

- Lie on your back, bend your knees, and place the roller under the balls of your feet. Reach your arms long by your side.
- Keeping the roller stable, inhale as you start to roll up your spine one vertebra at a time while scooping your belly.
- Exhale up to a neutral spine bridge position.
- Slowly lower yourself back down to the starting position, taking a full round of breath to get there.

Repeat this movement eight times.

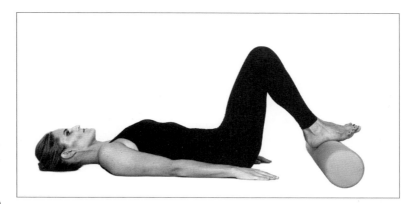

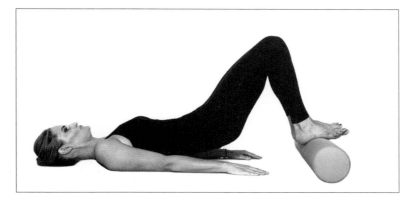

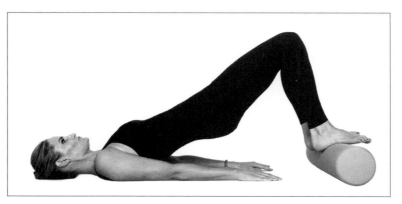

Figure Four

- Sit on the roller and reach your right arm behind you with your right hand on the mat, thumb out to the side. Cross your right ankle over your left knee in a figure four position. Press your left hand down into your right inner thigh.

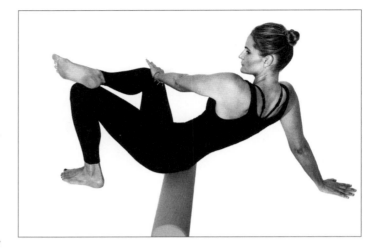

- Shift your weight slightly over to the left hip/glute area and roll back and forth a few inches in each direction.
- Next, roll in circles to help increase circulation and blood flow and to reduce congestion.

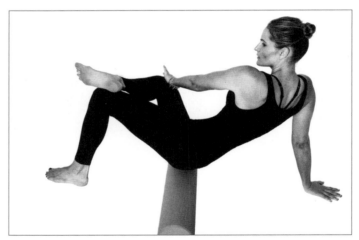

Repeat this movement on the other side.

Figure Four Circular Roll

- Sit on the roller and cross your right leg over your left knee to form a figure four.
- Lean to the right so the pressure of the roller hits all of your glute, and roll in a circular motion around your tush, forward and back.

Repeat this movement eight times on each side, alternating sides.

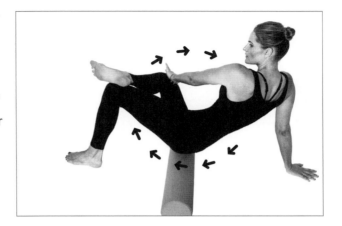

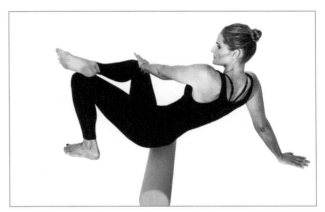

Glute Roll

- Sit down on your mat with the roller placed beneath your tush. Place your hands behind you on the mat. Bring your knees and feet together and lift your heels up so only your toes are touching the mat.
- Lean to the left side of your tush (including your knees), and roll from the inside to the outside of your tush so that you are massaging the entire side of the booty from the sacrum to the greater trochanter bones of the outer hip.

Complete this movement on each side for about thirty seconds per side.

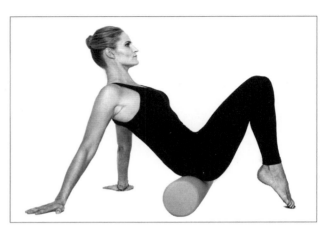

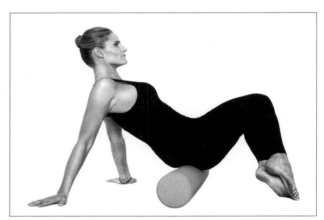

High Frog

- Press the soles of your feet together so that your knees are bent out to the sides, and place the sides of your ankles on the roller.
- Inhale and press your pubic bone up to the ceiling, engaging your core and keeping the roller stable.
- Exhale as you lower and hover your hips over the mat.

Repeat this movement five to eight times.

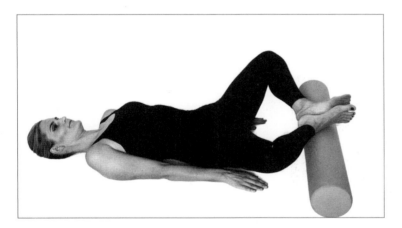

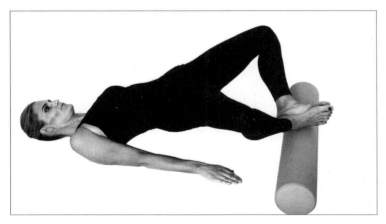

Inverted Figure Four Circles

- Lie down on the mat and come to a bridge position, sliding the roller under your hips/sacrum. Hold either end of the roller to stabilize yourself. Bend and lift your knees, and then cross your right ankle over your left knee, creating an inverted figure four.
- Inhale as you roll to the right while keeping your ribs and shoulders stable.
- Exhale as you circle down and back around up to the starting position.

Repeat this motion five times on each side, alternating sides.

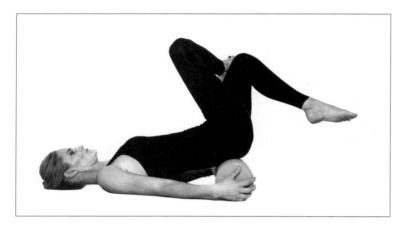

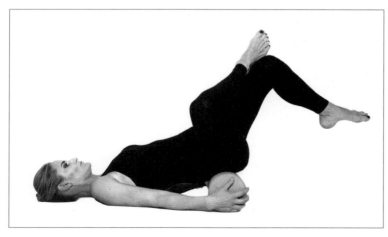

Inverted Tush Roll

- Slide the roller under your hips/sacrum (the triangular bone at the base of your spine), just above the tailbone. Lift your knees up so they are hovering directly over your hips. Hold either side of the roller.
- Inhale as you twist and draw your knees over to the left at a 45-degree angle.
- Exhale, using your core to return to center.

Repeat this movement eight times on each side, alternating sides.

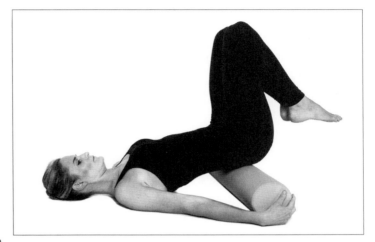

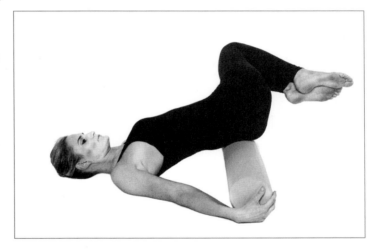

Kneeling Side Crab

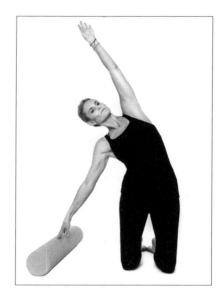

- Come to a kneeling position and place the roller to the right of your body. Stretch your left hand up toward the ceiling and exhale as you bend your entire body over to the right until the palm of your right hand comes down to the roller at your side.

- Hold this position as you bend your left arm behind your head, reach your left leg out to the side, and bend the knee to tone your outer tush. Inhale as you lift your left knee up to the ceiling while keeping your upper body, hips, and the roller stable.

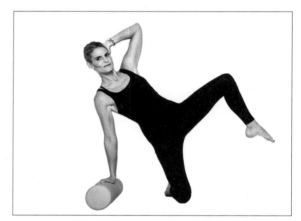

- Exhale as you lower your top knee down, keeping the foot and ankle stable.

Repeat this movement eight times, then repeat on the other side.

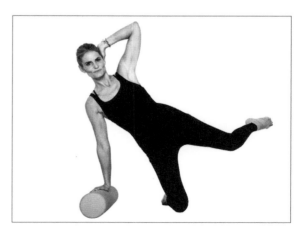

Roller Bridge Walk

- Lie on your back, reaching your arms long by your side, with your knees bent and feet placed on the mat hip width apart, about a foot away from your tush. Place the foam roller under the arches of your feet. Engaging your glutes, hamstrings, and core, press into your arms as you lift your hips up toward the ceiling so that your body forms a straight diagonal line from your knees and your shoulders.

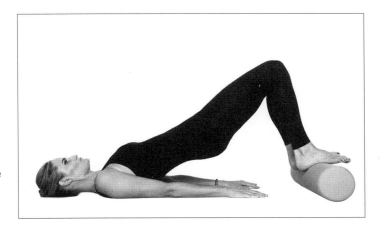

- Keeping your right knee bent, inhale as you lift your right foot and stabilize the roller with your left foot.
- Exhale as you return your right foot to the roller. Repeat the exercise with your left leg.

Repeat this movement eight times each side, alternating sides.

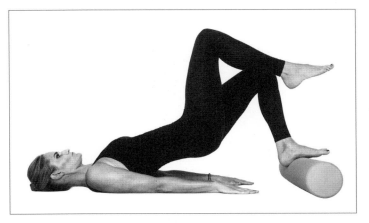

Single-Leg Squat Kick

- Stand with your feet hip width apart and reach your arms out to the side, with palms down.
- Inhale as you lean into your right foot and lift and reach your left foot up off the mat.
- Exhale as you bend your right knee and come back to center, returning your left foot to the mat.

Repeat this movement ten times per side, alternating sides.

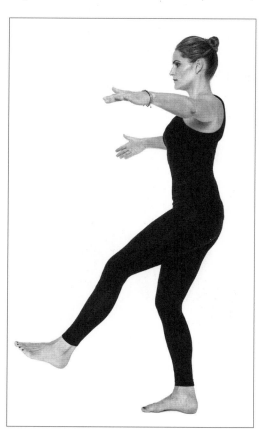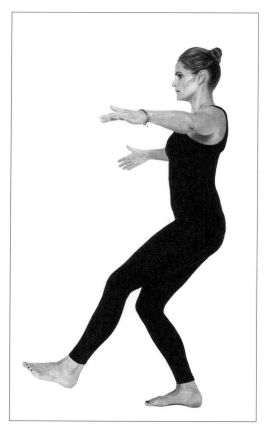

HIPS

Crisscross Backbend

- Sit up tall with your ankles crossed, knees wide. Place the roller about six inches behind you and press your palms into the roller, thumbs out to the side.
- Inhale as you press your palms into the roller to lift up and press your pubic bone forward, gazing up as you lift through your chest.
- Exhale as you release back down to the starting position.

Repeat this movement eight to ten times.Switch the leg cross and repeat five times on the other side.

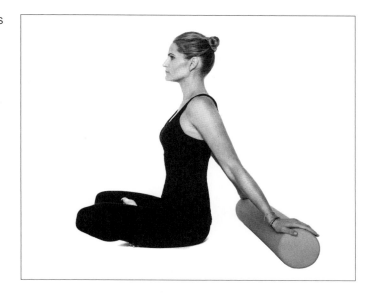

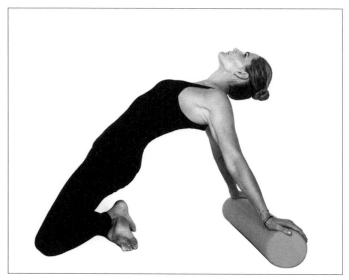

Side of Hip Roll

- Sit down with one hip placed on the mat. Prop yourself up by grounding your lower hand on the mat with your wrist crease directly under your shoulder. Place the roller under your seated hip, edging it toward your outer hip. Bend your top leg to ground your foot down in front of the extended leg for support and leverage.
- Use your grounded hand and upper leg to move the roller a few inches up and down the outer hip and thigh, stopping just above the knee. Exhale deeply as you draw in and inhale as you extend.

Repeat this movement on each side eight to ten times.

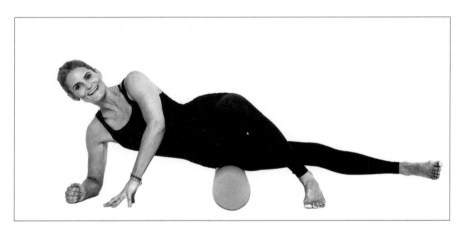

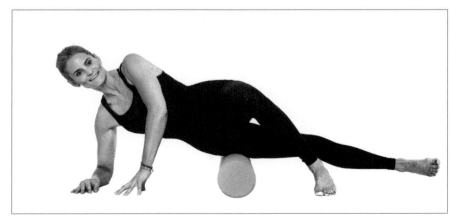

Front of Hip Roll

- Lie facedown on the mat and place the roller under your left thigh. Prop yourself up so that you are supporting your weight with your left forearm and right palm.
- Roll your weight slightly over to the left. Inhale as you roll the few inches along the front of your upper thigh to your hip, and exhale as you roll back down to the upper thigh. Repeat this movement eight times; then repeat on the other side.

Repeat this movement eight times, then repeat on alternate side.

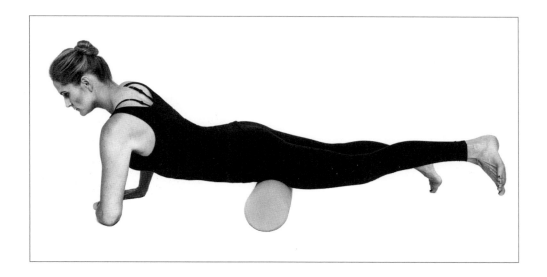

Internal and External TFL Roll

- Place the area right above the bony part of your right hip and below your pelvis on the roller, taking care not to place the roller directly on your hip joint. This will target the tensor fasciae latae (TFL), a muscle that runs from the hip to the top of the pelvis. You will not have to roll much with this move as it covers a small surface area. Cross your left leg over your right, grounding down through your left foot.
- Inhale and exhale long and smooth as you use your left foot to create motion and roll up and down this small area eight to ten times.
- Internally rotate your foot and knee to roll the outer side of your TFL, again for eight to ten times.
- Externally rotate your feet and knees to roll the more medial side of your TFL, again for eight to ten times.

Repeat each of the three variations of this movement eight to ten times.

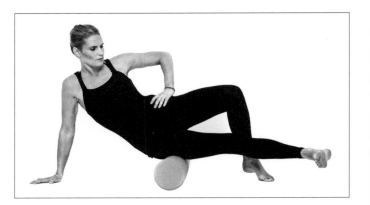

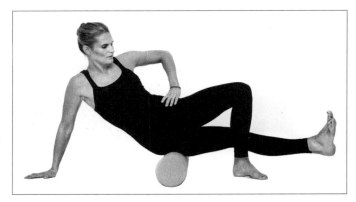

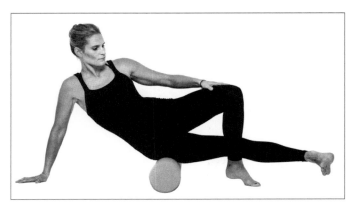

Kneeling Side Kicks

- Come to a kneeling position and place the roller to the right of your body. Reach your left arm up and exhale as you bend your entire body over to the right side until the palm of your right hand comes down to the roller at your side.
- Hold this position as you extend your left leg long and slightly in front of you.
- Inhale as you reach your left arm toward your right shin, keeping the roller stable. Exhale as you reach your left leg back and your left arm back in extension while bending the knee. Inhale as you reach your arm and leg forward. Exhale as you reach back.

Repeat this movement eight to ten times, then repeat on the other side.

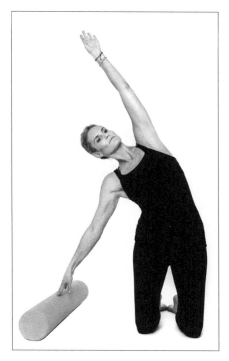

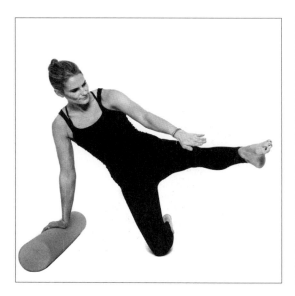

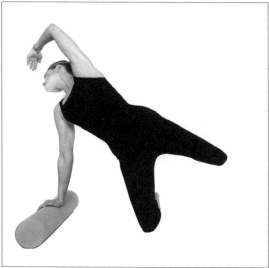

Psoas Backbend Twist

- Come down to your knees and place the roller directly behind you. Bring your right hand as close as you can get it to the middle of the roller behind you, and lift your left arm up to the ceiling. Lift your hips up and forward.
- Keeping the roller stable, inhale as you begin lowering your hips and your left arm down in front of you.
- Exhale as you press your hips forward and up, lift your deep core muscles up, and return to the starting position.

Repeat this motion eight times on each side.

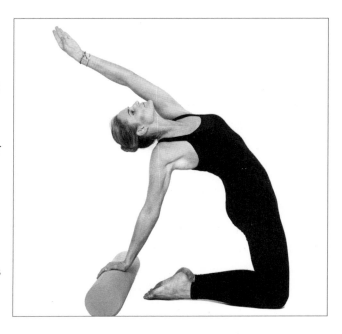

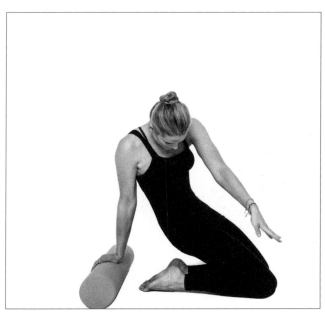

Psoas De-Bunch

- Lie on the mat faceup, with the roller placed under your sacrum. Bend one knee and draw it into your chest. Keep the other leg extended down on the mat in front of you, flexing and reaching through the heel.
- As you inhale, lift your extended leg two inches off the mat. Hold here for three slow, full breaths, allowing your hips to fully extend and elongate. After your third round of breath, exhale as you release your extended leg down to the mat, reaching through your flexed heel.

Repeat this movement eight to ten times on each side.

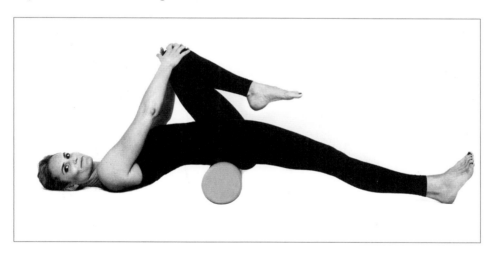

Roller-Supported Jackknife

• Lie down on your back on the mat, bend your knees, and place your feet down on the mat, hip width apart. Lift your hips up off the mat and slide the roller under your hips and sacrum, just above the tailbone. Lift your knees up directly over your hips and then extend your legs straight up to the ceiling. Bend your elbows out to the side to anchor your upper body firmly on the mat and press your palms into the roller.

• Inhale as you lower your legs to a 45-degree angle, keeping your belly drawn in.

• Keeping your core, hamstrings, and arms active the entire time, exhale as you roll your spine and hips over your head until your legs are parallel to the floor.

• Exhale as you reach your legs to a 45-degree angle.

• Inhale again as you begin to roll yourself back down with control, one vertebra at a time. Exhale to come all the way down, returning your hips and sacrum to the roller.

Repeat this movement eight times.

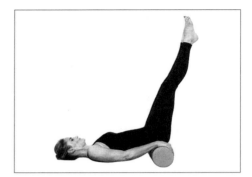

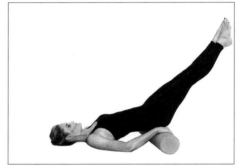

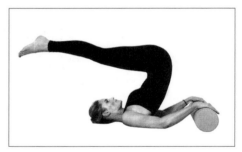

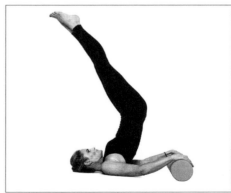

Rolling Lunge

- Stand on your right foot with your right knee slightly bent, and put the top of your left foot on the foam roller behind you with your back leg straight. Raise your arms directly overhead.
- Inhale as you bend your right knee, keeping the knee over the heel, and extend your left hip and leg back, pressing into the foam roller as it rolls up your shin until your right thigh is nearly parallel to the floor.
- Exhale as you use your deep core to pull yourself back up to the starting position.

Repeat this movement eight times on each side.

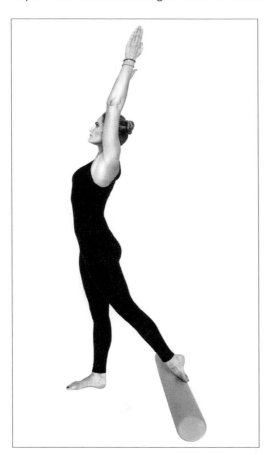
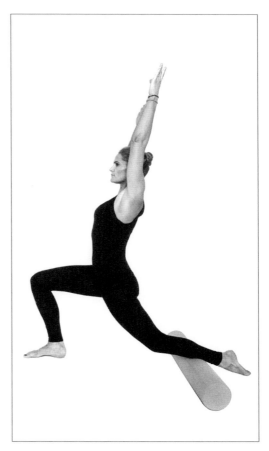

Standing Hip Circles

- Stand with your feet hip width apart, a tall neutral spine, and soft knees.
- Imagine that you are using your hips to draw large circles on a piece of paper. Inhale as you shift your hips over to the right and then circle them to the front.
- Exhale as you slide your hips to the left and finish by circling them to the back. The movement should be fluid and smooth throughout.

Repeat this movement eight to ten times, in both directions, moving in a fluid circle.

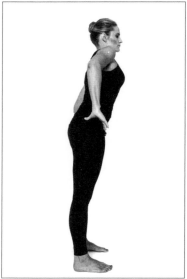
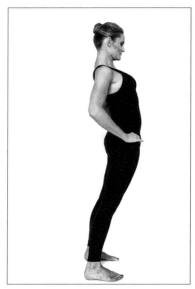
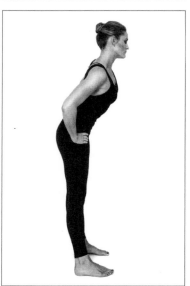
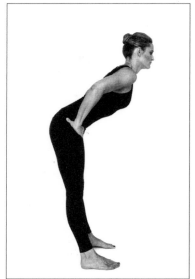

TFL Roll

- Lie on your right side with the roller placed just above the hip joint (*not* on the hip joint) and below the pelvis. You're going to target the tensor fasciae latae (TFL), which is the muscle that runs from your hip to the top of your pelvis. You will not have to roll much with this exercise, as it is a small surface area.
- Inhale and exhale as you roll up and down this small area.

Repeat this movement eight to ten times on each side.

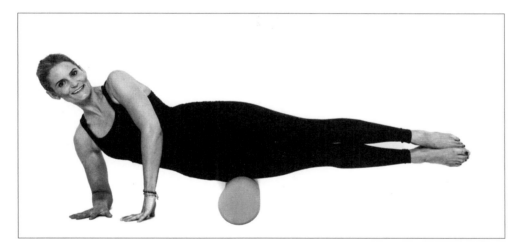

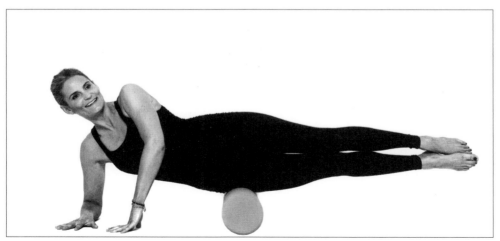

LOWER LEGS

Calf Roll

- Sit on your mat with your legs close together and the roller placed under both of your calves, right below the knee joint. Place your hands palms-down on the floor a few inches out from either side of your hips, fingers pointing outward. Press down into your hands to lift your bottom off the mat, keeping your calves balanced on the roller. Make sure to draw your shoulders down and back to avoid hunching.
- Continue pressing your hands down and engage your core, exhaling to slowly drive your body weight forward so that the roller stops right above the ankle.
- As you inhale, slowly draw the roller back so that it stops right below the knee.

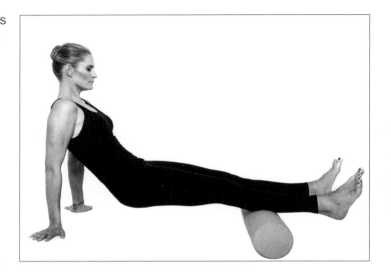

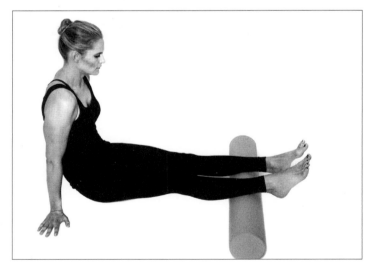

Repeat three sets of eight rolls. The roller should be placed under the center of your calves for the first set, the inner edge of the calves for the second set, and the outer edge of the calves for the third set.

Calf Roll with Rotations

- Sit on your mat with your legs close together and the roller placed under both of your calves, right below the knee joint. Place your hands palms-down on the floor a few inches out from either side of your hips, fingers pointing outward. Press down into your hands to lift your bottom off the mat, keeping your calves balanced on the roller. Make sure to draw your shoulders down and back to avoid hunching.

- Continue pressing your hands down and engage your core, exhaling as you slowly drive your body weight forward so that the roller stops right above the ankle.

- After you've finished rolling down the center of your calves, internally rotate your feet (turn them inward) and repeat this rolling motion, this time rolling through the inner part of the calf.

- Externally rotate the feet (turn them outward) and roll, this time along the outer part of the calves.

- Return to parallel and release yourself back to the floor.

Repeat this movement eight times per variation.

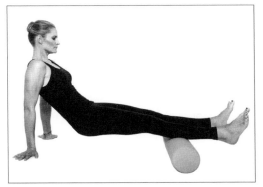

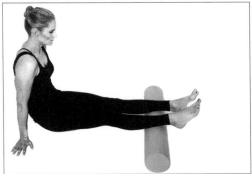

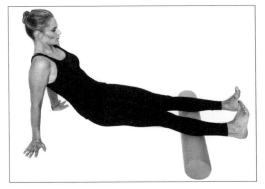

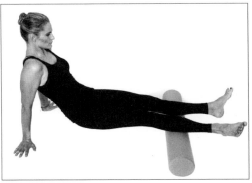

Core Stability Footwork

- Lie on the roller with a neutral spine, with the roller supporting you from head to tailbone. Place your forearms on either side of the roller to stabilize. Lift your legs with your knees bent at a 90-degree angle, heels together, toes apart.
- Lift your shoulder blades off the roller and curl up over your bra line, keeping a long neck.
- Maintaining your curl, inhale as you slowly extend your legs out to a 45-degree angle, maintaining a neutral spine.
- Exhale as you slowly draw your legs back in to return to the starting position.

Repeat this movement eight to ten times.

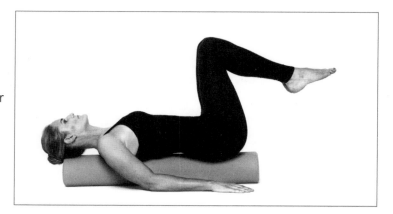

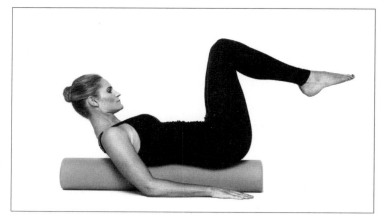

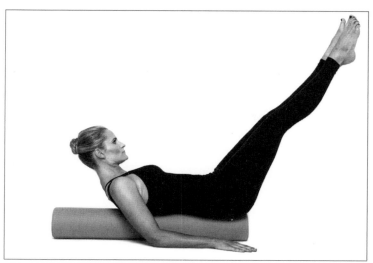

Foot Roll

- Place the ball of your left foot on the roller six inches in front of your standing foot while balancing on your right foot.
- Inhale as you press your foot into the roller, moving the roller from your arch to the front of your heel. Apply as much pressure as you can, to the point where you feel that hurts-so-good sensation.
- Exhale and roll back to your starting position.

Repeat three sets of eight rolls on each side. The roller should be placed under the center of the arch.

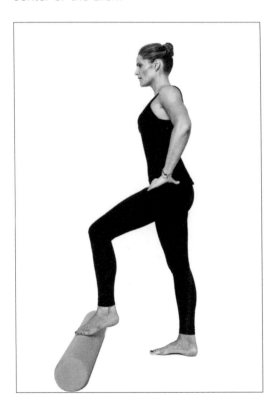
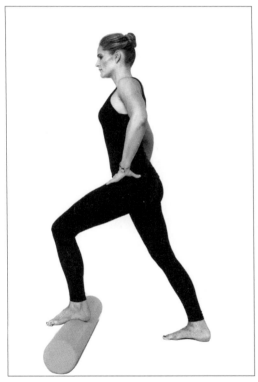

Heel Lifts

• Stand with your feet hip width apart and arms raised overhead.

• As you inhale, pull your belly in and up as you slowly lift your heels off the floor, keeping your ankles stable.

• Exhale as you slowly lower your heels back down to the floor.

Repeat this movement eight times.

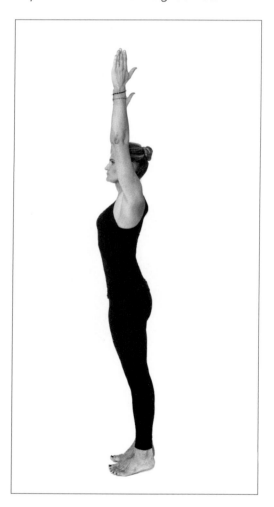
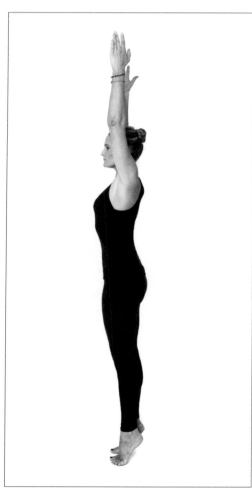

Kneeling Lunge Shin Roll

- Come to a kneeling lunge on your mat, beginning with your right leg forward and bent at a 90-degree angle. Place the roller just below the kneecap of your left leg. Place your hands slightly in front of your shoulders on either side of your foot.

- Inhale as you ground through your front foot and pull yourself forward, straightening your back leg as the roller rolls down your shin.

- Exhale as you return to the starting position.

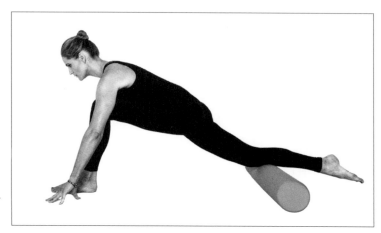

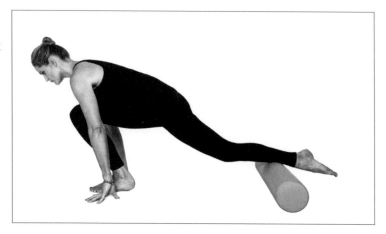

Repeat this movement eight to ten times per leg.

Standing Footwork

- Stand with your feet turned out. Stand the roller up in front of you and place both of your hands on top of the roller for a little bit of support.
- Lift your heels so that you're standing on your toes. Keep weight even through all five toes of each foo (don't collapse inward or outward).
- Keeping your heels lifted, ankles stable, and spine neutral, inhale as you bend your knees wide and lower down a few inches.
- Continue to keep your heels lifted as you exhale and straighten your knees (without locking them), returning to the starting position.

Repeat this movement eight times.

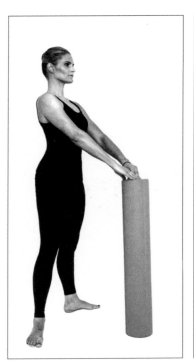 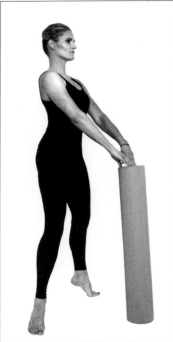 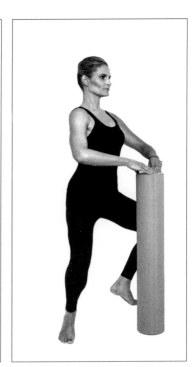

Standing Stability

- Come to stand on the foam roller with the arches of your feet at the center of the roller, aligning your body's center of gravity over your feet. Find your neutral spine and maintain a slight soft bend in your knees as you balance on the roller.
- For stability and support, hold on to a nearby wall, chair, or counter.

Continue this balance work for one to two minutes, getting back on the roller when (and if!) you lose your balance.

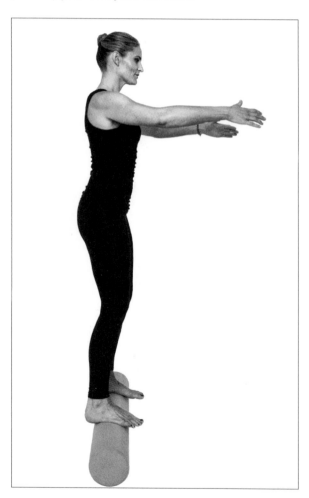

Tennis Ball Arch Roll

- Stand next to a wall or sturdy chair where you can steady yourself and place a tennis ball under the heel of your left foot.
- Roll the ball back and forth from your heel to your toes for 30 seconds; then switch feet. Start with a softer pressure for your first round. Then gradually apply a bit more weight as you go deeper into the fascia and mobilize your feet.

Repeat this movement four times on each side, alternating sides.

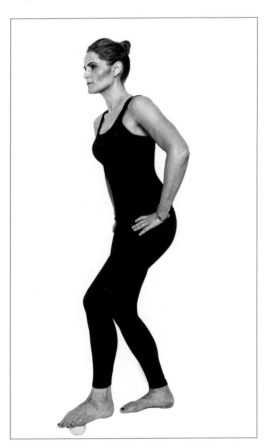
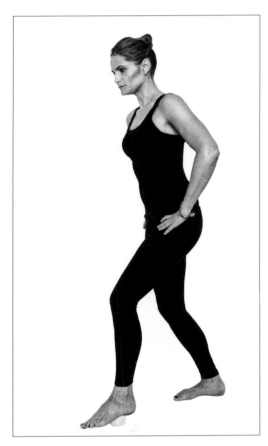

Toe Tendon/Joint Mobilization

- Come down to a deep squat position. Shift the roller under your mid-upper shins and keep your toes curled under and forward, with toes spread wide and heels reaching back so that your feet are really stretched out. Keep your elbows soft and place your hands shoulder-width apart on the mat. Keep your shoulders drawn down for the duration of the exercise.
- Use your feet to roll forward and back, stretching your feet and rolling your shins.

Repeat this movement eight times.

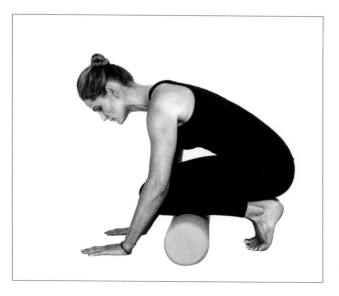

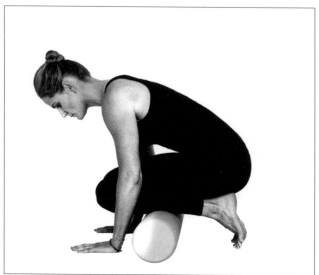

THIGHS

Back of Thigh Roll

- Sit on your mat with the roller under your hamstrings, right above the knee joint. Place your hands on the mat behind you, with fingertips slightly turned out. Press your hands into the mat to lift your bottom off the floor, and engage your core.
- Keep your shoulders back and inhale as you roll the roller up the back of your thighs.
- Exhale as you roll back down to the starting position.

Repeat this movement eight to ten times.

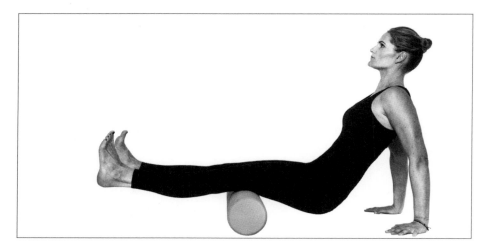

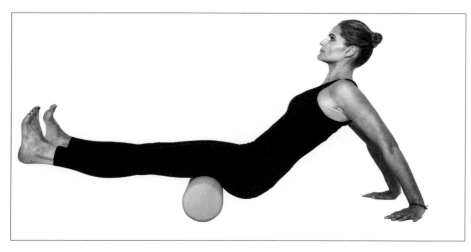

Chair Pose

- Come to a standing position with your feet and thighs pressed together. Reach your arms up to the ceiling with palms facing in toward each other.
- Inhale as you bend your knees as if you're going to sit down in a chair. Keeping your weight equally balanced between both feet, activate your entire foot by spreading your toes and pressing into your pinkie toes, big toes, and heels. Stay in this position for twenty seconds, inhaling and exhaling deeply while holding this pose.

Repeat this movement five times.

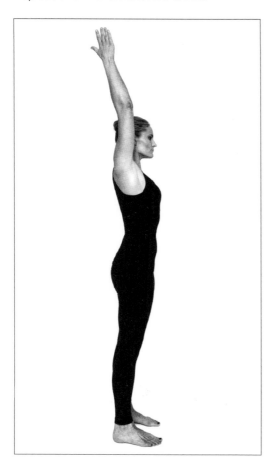 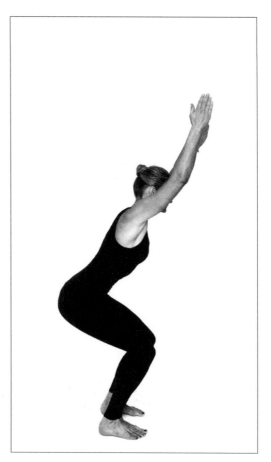

Front of Thigh Roll

• Place the roller above the knees. Bring your elbows to the mat about two inches behind your shoulders and make fists. Engage your core to prop yourself up and protect your lower back.
• Using your arms and core, exhale as you pull yourself forward as the roller rolls up the front of your thighs.
• Inhale as you press the roller down to just above the front of your knees.

Repeat this movement eight to ten times.

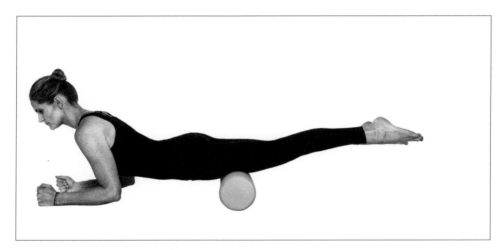

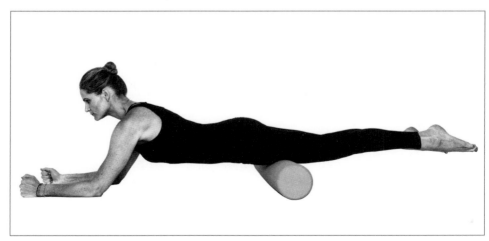

Goddess Pose Roll

- Place the roller under your hips, with your feet together and knees wide. Keep your belly engaged to prevent overarching your lower back. Come down to your forearms with your belly facing the mat.
- Exhale as you roll all the way down to your inner knees.
- Inhale as you roll up to your pubic bone attachment.

Repeat this movement eight times.

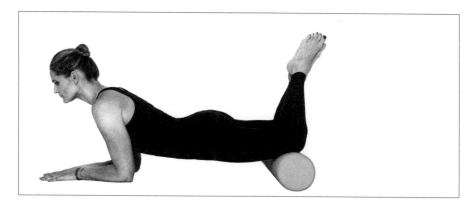

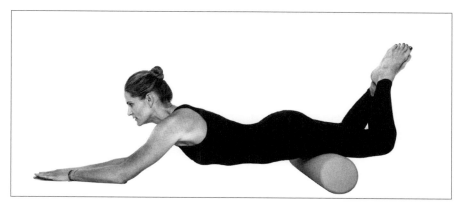

Inner Thigh Cross

- Sit on the roller and reach your arms behind you, legs stretched in front of you. Plant your palms down on the mat with fingers facing outward. Keeping your core engaged, lift both of your legs up to a 45-degree angle, heels together, toes apart.
- Inhale and exhale to lower your legs down a few inches.
- Continue to breathe slowly and steadily as you cross one leg over the other, alternating legs ten times.

Repeat this movement ten times.

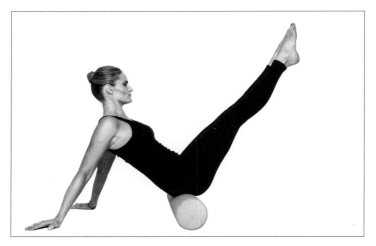

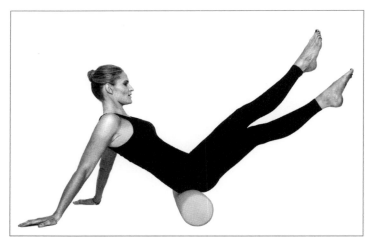

Inner Thigh Roll

- Come down to your forearms with your torso facing the mat, and place the roller under your right upper inner thigh. To do this, you will need to bend your right knee up and out to the side and place the foam roller up and under your groin.
- Taking care to keep your upper body square to the floor as you move, use your forearms and left leg to power the motion as you roll the roller down toward the knee (stopping just above it) and back up again.

Repeat this motion six to eight times on each side.

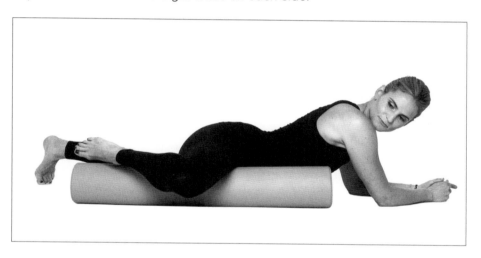

Lateral Lunge

- Stand on your mat with your feet spread into a straddle position, about three to four feet apart. Stand the roller up vertically on the floor in front of you.
- Place your hands on top of the roller, with arms extended and spine straight.
- Inhale as you lean to the right, bending your right leg and straightening your left leg. Exhale as you hold the stretch.
- Repeat this motion on the other side.

Repeat this movement five times on each side.

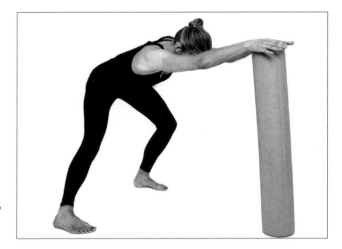

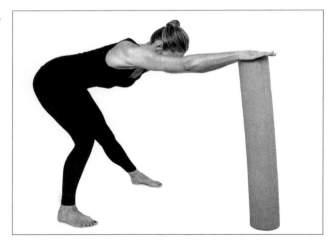

Low Lunge with Thigh Extension

- Come to the mat in a bent knee lunge, beginning with your right foot forward, knee stacked directly over your ankle at a 90-degree angle. Place your left leg behind you with the top of your foot flat on the mat. Slowly lift your core and left arm up, keeping your shoul-ders relaxed as you twist your body to the right and reach around to the back of your left thigh to feel the front of your hip and psoas stretch and lengthen while you breathe into it.

- Gently deepen into the stretch for about thirty seconds as you continue to breathe slowly and steadily. This movement will allow you to go deeper and send oxygenated blood to the hips.

Repeat this movement on the other side.

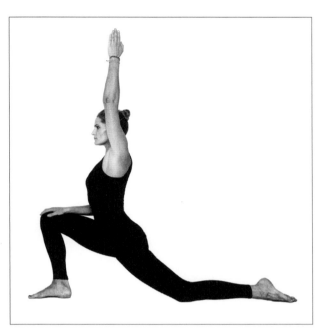

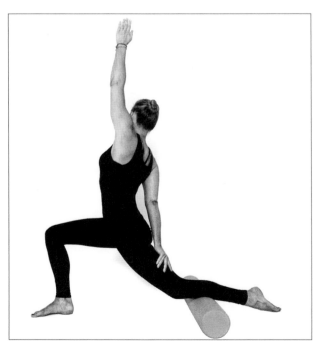

Outer Thigh Roll

- Lie down on your right side, placing the roller under the upper outside of your right thigh. Bend your left knee and cross your left leg over your right, placing your left foot flat on the floor in front of your right knee. Bring your right forearm down to the mat to ground you.

- Use your left foot and right forearm to roll the length of your iliotibial band (IT band) along the roller from your hip all the way down to just above your knee joint. (The IT band is the thick line of fascia that runs along the outside of your body, from your pelvis all the way down to just below your knee.) As you get closer to your knee, you may feel more tenderness, so be prepared to use your left arm and foot to ease the pressure. The more weight you bear in your foot, the less you will place on your IT band.

Repeat this motion eight times, then repeat on the other side.

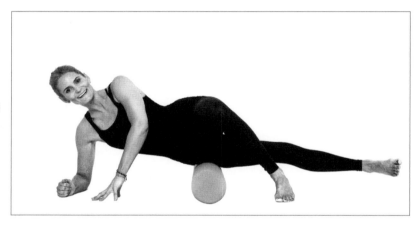

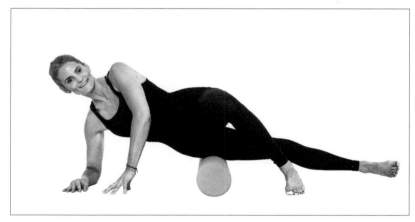

Pigeon Inner Thigh Roll

- Place the roller about a foot in front of you and come down to your knees. Bring your right leg in front of the roller so that your right calf is parallel to the roller, and lean forward into a pigeon hip stretch, so that the roller is now at the inner edge of your sitz bone. Use your front foot to keep the roller stable and lift up into a tall spine. Keep your left leg long and straight back behind the roller.
- Breathing steadily, slowly roll front and back to smooth out the inner thigh and pelvic floor attachment.

Repeat this movement eight times on each side, alternating sides.

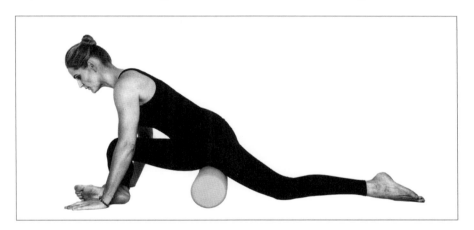

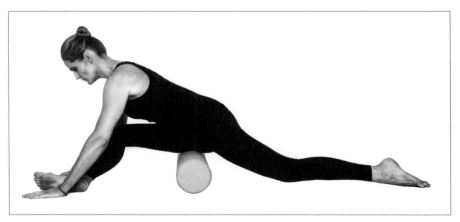

Rolling Bridge Heel Pulls

- Lie on your back, bend your knees, and place the roller under the balls of your feet. Reach your arms long by your side.
- Inhale as you start to roll your spine up one vertebra at a time and exhale all the way up until you're in a bridge position.
- Inhale again as you pull the roller an inch toward you and then exhale as you push the roller back one inch. Repeat this movement as a pulsation eight times.
- Exhale as you roll your spine down one vertebra at a time and extend your legs in front of you.

Repeat the pulling portion of this movement eight times.

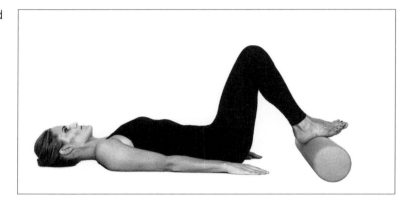

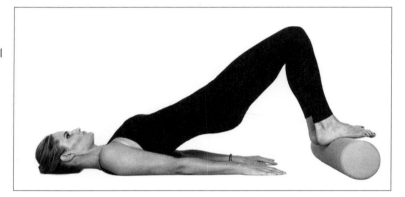

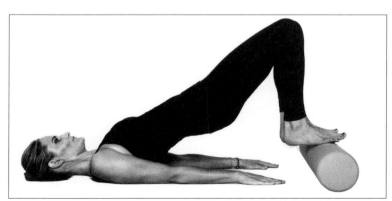

Rolling Leg Pull Front

- Place the roller under your hands and come to a push-up or plank position. Reach your heels back, spreading your toes and really stretching the feet and arches while simultaneously engaging your entire core and arms.

- Inhale as you shift your weight forward onto your toes while lifting your heels as the roller moves forward and your abs kick in even more.

- Exhale as you reach your heels back to stretch your feet and activate your core while using your abs and feet to press the roller back.

Repeat this movement ten times.

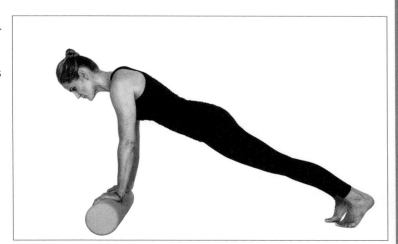

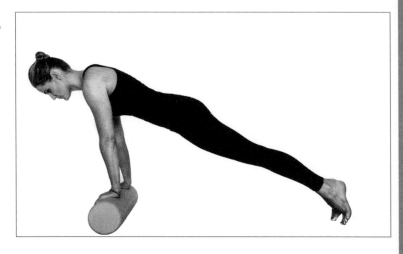

Seated Single-Leg Circle

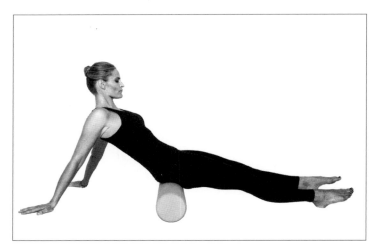

- Sit on the roller and reach your arms behind you, chest and heart open, legs stretched in front of you and the back of your heels resting on the mat. Plant your palms down on the mat with fingers facing outward.

- Lift your right leg to a 45-degree angle. Keeping your breath smooth and your belly engaged, move your leg in a clockwise direction to make six slow, controlled circles. Repeat this movement six times on the left side.

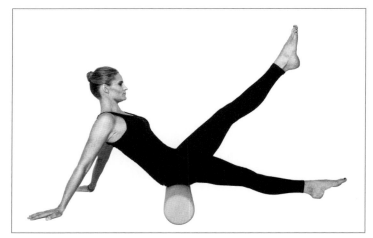

- Lift your right leg so that it is elevated from the mat and repeat this same motion six times, but this time in a counterclockwise direction. Repeat this movement six times on the left side.

Repeat this movement six times on each side and in each direction, alternating sides.

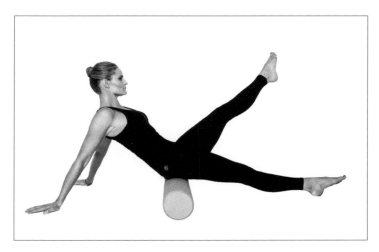

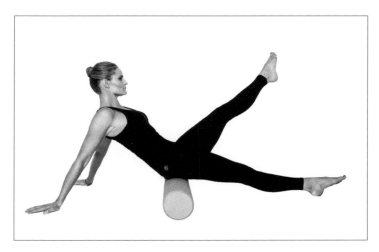

Sexy Cat

- Bring the roller in front of you and place your arms on it, right below the elbow joints. Reach your sitz bones up and your chest down, feel your sitz bones opening like a flower blooming.
- Keeping the roller stable, inhale as you lean your hips over to the left.
- Exhale as you lean your hips over to the right.

Repeat this movement six times on each side, alternating directions.

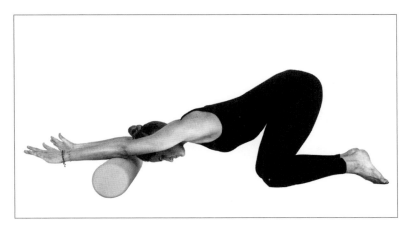

Side Kicks/Inner Thigh Lifts

- Bring your right hip down to the mat and place the roller under your right side at your waistline. Place your right elbow directly under your right shoulder joint. Bend your top knee and bring the heel of your top foot in front of you, with your knee facing up to the ceiling. Straighten your bottom leg.
- Inhale as you use your inner thigh to lift the lower leg, keeping your upper body and the roller stable.
- Exhale as you lower your bottom leg down to the mat.

Repeat this motion eight times on each side.

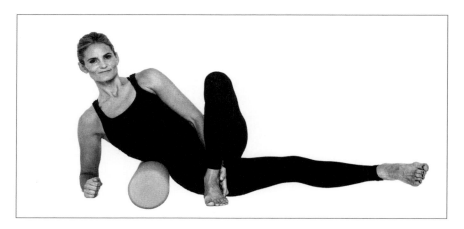

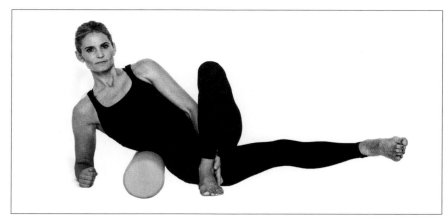

Sitz Bone Roll

- Place the roller on the mat and sit on it so that your sitz bones are directly on the roller.
- Extend your right leg long and roll the roller approximately two inches in each direction as you keep your breath smooth and long. This motion will reduce density where your adductors and hamstrings attach to your pelvis.

Continue this movement for thirty seconds, then switch to the other side.

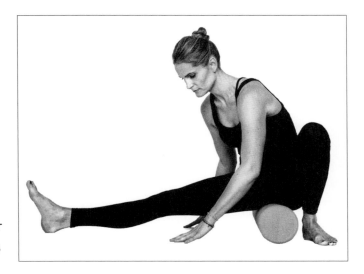

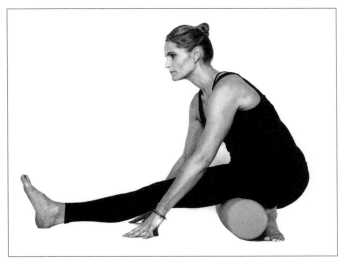

Stomach Massage

- Sit up tall on the mat with your knees bent, heels together, and toes apart. Place your toes on the roller and engage your core, thighs, and arms. Reach your arms out to a 45-degree angle, keeping your shoulder blades drawn down toward your hips. (In other words, don't hunch your neck—it should feel nice and long, not scrunched up.)
- Engage your arm muscles and inhale as you extend your legs long, pressing the roller away from you and simultaneously rolling your spine into a C-shape while pulling your belly in and up.
- As you exhale, engage your core and draw the roller back in to the point where your knees are bent and your spine is tall.

Repeat this exercise eight to ten times.

Thigh Stretch

- Kneel on the mat with your knees hip width apart, big toes together. Bring the roller over your head, placing a hand on either side of it. Keep your shoulders down and chest open. Establish a neutral spine (see box on page 20), and maintain a stable spine and pelvis throughout this exercise.
- As you inhale, begin hinging back from your knee joints. Engage your inner thighs and pull your belly in and up to keep the weight off your knees. Hold the pose for three seconds.
- Exhale as you press your shins down and slowly float back up to your starting position.

Repeat this movement eight to ten times.

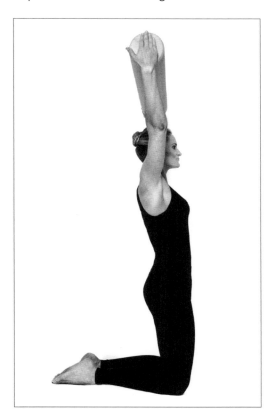
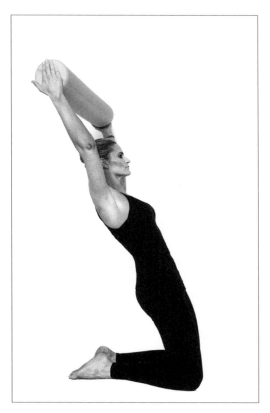

Thigh Stretch Twist

- Kneel on the mat with your knees hip width apart, big toes together. Bring the roller over your head, placing a hand on either side of it. Keep your shoulders down and chest open. Establish a neutral spine (see the box on page 20) and maintain a stable spine and pelvis throughout this exercise.
- As you inhale, begin hinging back from your knee joints. Engage your inner thighs and pull your belly in and up to keep the weight off your knees and press your shins down into the floor.
- Exhale and twist your entire body to the right.
- Inhale back to center and exhale to the left.
- Inhale to return to center and exhale back up to the starting position.

Repeat this movement five times on each side, alternating sides.

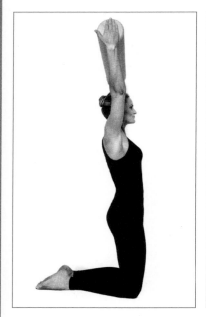
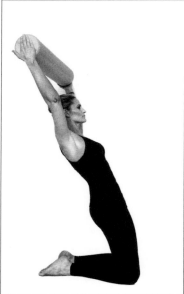
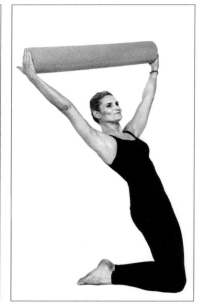

Arm Circles

- Lie on the roller the long way, so that your entire spine is supported from head to tailbone. Reach your arms out to the side in a T-shape with the palms of your hands facing up to open and expand the chest.
- Inhale deeply expanding your lungs as you reach your arms up overhead while keeping them parallel to the floor.
- Exhale as you draw your arms up to the ceiling and back down by your hips.

Repeat this movement eight times.

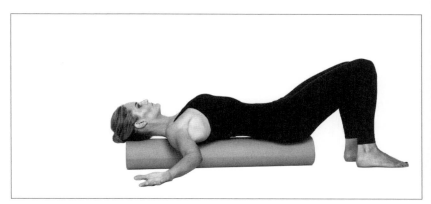

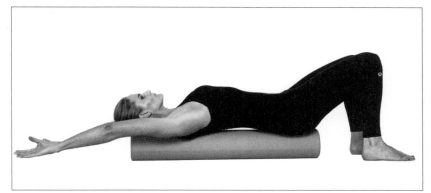

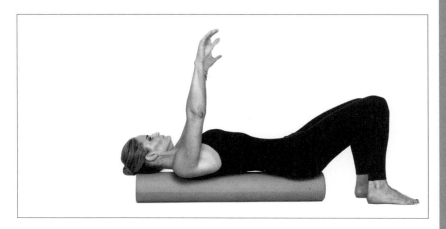

Collarbone Alignment

- Place the roller behind your upper back with your elbows bent and palms up. Bend your knees and plant your feet on the floor together.
- Exhale as you simultaneously lower your knees to the left and look to the right. Inhale to lift back to center and then exhale as you lower your knees to the right and look to the left. Inhale to lift back to center.

Repeat this movement eight times to each side.

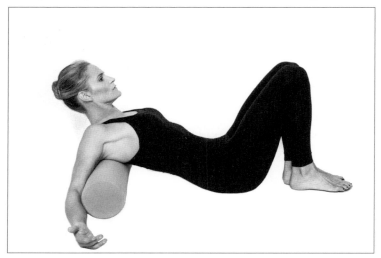

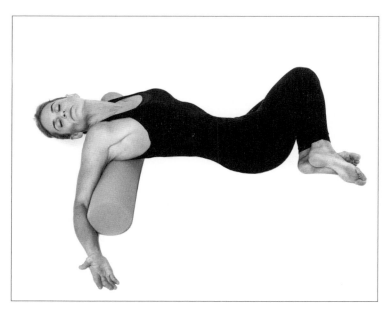

Neck Massage

- Lie down on your back and place the roller at the base of your skull, putting your hands on either end to stretch the arms and keep it steady.
- Inhale and turn your head to the left, feeling the roller gently massage your neck.
- Exhale as you come back to center.
- Inhale to fully rotate your neck to the right. Exhale as you return to center.

Repeat this movement eight times on each side.

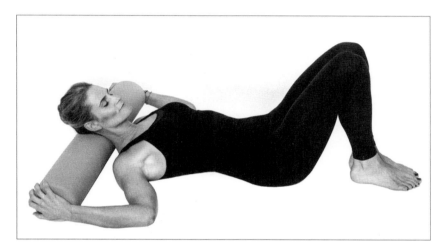

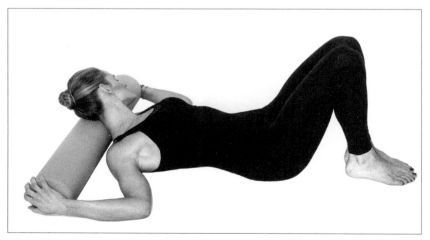

Rolling Swan with Neck Twist

- Lie belly-down on the mat, with arms long in front of you and the roller placed just below your elbow joints, thumbs facing up. Reach your heels away from your heart to feel oppositional energy and decompress your spine.

- Inhale and roll the roller toward you, extending your spine and lifting your heart as you roll your shoulders back (taking care to keep your glutes relaxed the entire time so you don't jam your lower back while lifting up). Exhale to come all the way up to the top, being sure to pull your abs up and in.

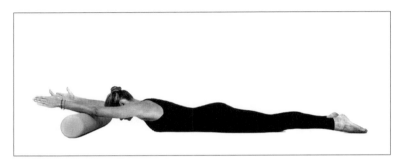

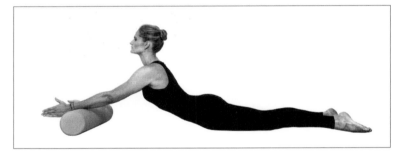

- While you are holding yourself up in extension, inhale and turn your head to the right. Exhale to return to center. Then turn to the left as you inhale. Exhale to return to center once again.

- Inhale as you begin to lower down, slowly resisting as you go; exhale as you come all the way down.

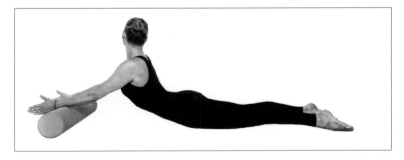

Repeat this movement eight times.

Roll Out the Kinks

- Lie on the mat with the roller placed under your back at the bra line, leaning your midback over the roller. Gently interlace your fingers behind your head to support your head and neck.
- Using your feet to drive the movement, inhale as you roll up to massage the upper back and shoulder blades, stopping at the top of the shoulder blades.
- Exhale as you roll and massage down the spine, stopping at the bottom of your rib cage. Be careful *not* to roll back and forth on the lower back because it can create too much pressure or force on your disks and vertebrae.

Repeat this movement eight to ten times.

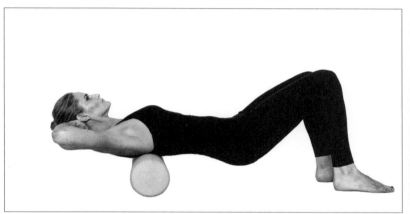

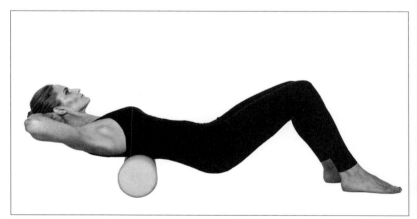

Snow Angels

- Lie on the roller with your spine supported from head to tailbone. Begin with your arms extended down by your sides, with the palms of your hands facing up to open and expand the chest.
- Inhale deeply as you reach your arms up overhead slowly and with control, keeping them as close to the mat as possible and parallel to the floor.
- Exhale completely as you draw your arms back down to your sides.

Repeat this movement eight times.

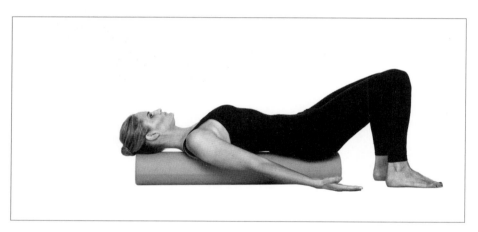

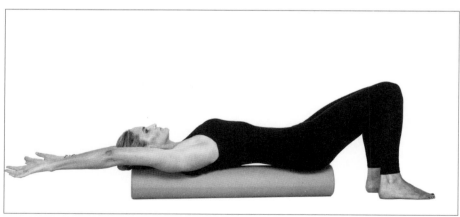

Upper Back Massage

- Lay the roller horizontally across the mat and lie back over it so that the roller is placed right beneath your shoulder blades (or at the bra line). Interlace your fingers and gently place your hands behind your head to support your neck and head.
- Place your feet on the floor hip width apart, knees bent up toward the ceiling. Using your feet to drive the move, inhale as you slowly roll the roller up to massage the upper back and shoulder blades. The more you breathe during this movement, the better, because oxygen nourishes the blood and tissues and also helps reduce stress.
- Exhale as you roll down, massaging the spine all the way down to the bottom of your rib cage. (Be careful *not* to roll back and forth on the lower back, because it can create too much pressure on your disks and vertebrae.)

Repeat this movement eight times.

Hourglass

- Place the roller under your left leg, just above the left anklebone, and cross your right leg over your left. Place your left elbow directly under your left shoulder, with your forearm flat on the floor and fingers spread; reach your right arm up and slightly back. Press down into your left leg and forearm, using this traction to lift your side body (or "hourglass") off the floor, taking care to keep the roller stable as you lift.
- Inhaling, resist as you lower your hips and right arm down, hovering a few inches above the mat.
- Exhale as you lift with your waist to return to your starting position.

Repeat this exercise eight to ten times before switching to the other side.

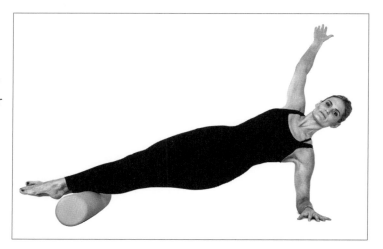

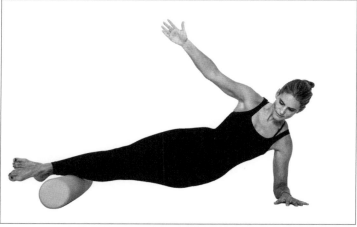

Hourglass with Arm Twist

- Place the roller under your left leg, just above the left anklebone, and cross your right leg over your left. Place your left elbow directly under your left shoulder, with your forearm flat on the floor and fingers spread; reach your right arm up and slightly back. Press down into your left leg and forearm, using this traction to lift your side body (or "hourglass") off the floor, taking care to keep the roller stable as you lift.

- Initiate the move with an inhale; exhale as you rotate your torso toward the left and reach your right arm under you to "thread the needle" while keeping your side body lifted. Follow your arm with your gaze by tucking your chin.

- Inhale as you lift your right arm back up to the starting position, again following it with your gaze as you move.

Repeat this movement eight to ten times, then repeat on the other side.

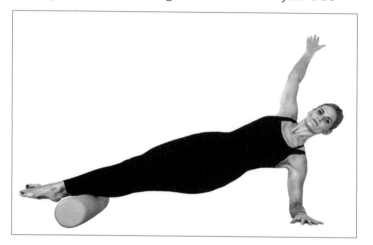

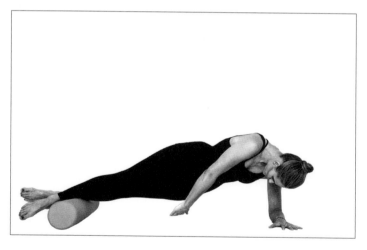

QL Roll

- Place the roller behind you.
- Come to a figure-four position with your left knee bent, right ankle crossed over your left thigh, right above the knee. Your forearms should be on the mat, palms on the roller, thumbs facing in. Lean your body to the right while feeling a subtle pressure on the right quadratus lumborum (QL), a lower back muscle between the bottom of your ribs and the top of your hips.
- Keeping the roller stable, press down into your foot while you inhale and curl your tailbone up; exhale and come back down.

Repeat this movement eight times on each side.

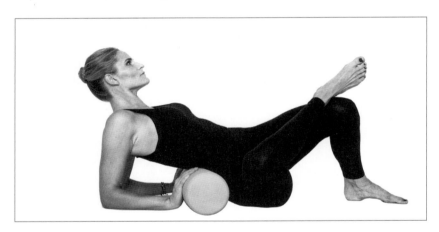

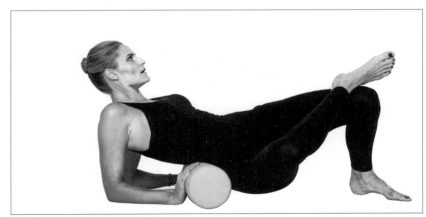

Roller CanCan Balance

- Sit on the roller with your arms reaching behind you, palms planted on the mat, and fingers pointed out to the sides. Keeping the roller stable, lift your knees up over your hips and engage your abs.
- Inhale as you roll your hips and knees over to the right, so that you're balancing on the roller with your right hip.
- Exhale and extend your legs out to a 45-degree angle, keeping your core connected.
- Inhale as you bend your knees back and turn so that your left hip is now balanced on the roller, repeating this motion from there.

Repeat this movement six times on each side, alternating sides.

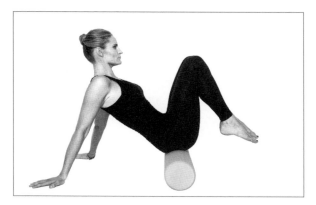

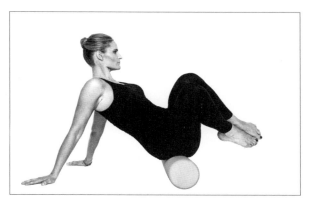

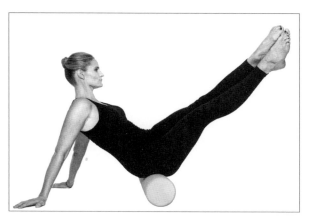

Roller Twist on Hip

- Lie on your right hip with your spine running parallel to the side of your mat and your legs hinged at a 45-degree angle toward the right front corner of the mat. Place the roller slightly below your right elbow joint.
- Inhale and gently press down into the roller to start rolling it to just above your wrist (this will tone your triceps and lats), while simultaneously lifting both legs up and rolling slightly to the left while balancing on your right tush and hip.
- Exhale at the top and hold while continuing to balance with the roller above your wrist.
- Inhale slowly to start reaching long as you come down and exhale all the way down to the mat as the roller returns to its starting position right below your elbow joint.

Repeat this movement eight times, then repeat on the other side.

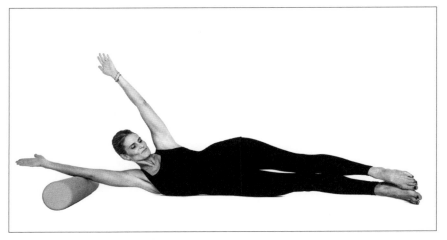

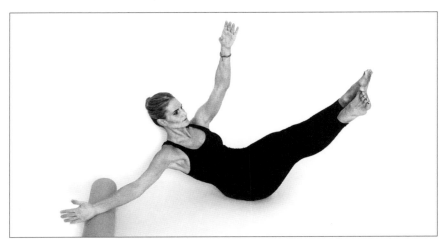

Rolling Mermaid Twist

- Place your right shin in front of you and your left shin out to the left side so that your knees are staggered. Place the roller to the right of you and put the palms of your hands on the roller. Reach and lift your sides and lift through the top of your head.

- Inhale as you roll the roller up your forearms to just below your elbows.

- Exhale as you roll back up to the starting position.

Repeat this movement five times, then repeat on the other side.

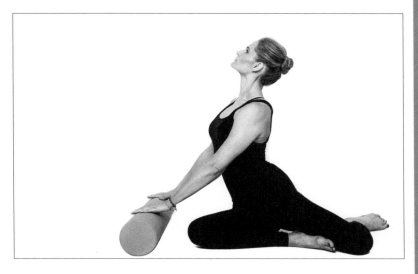

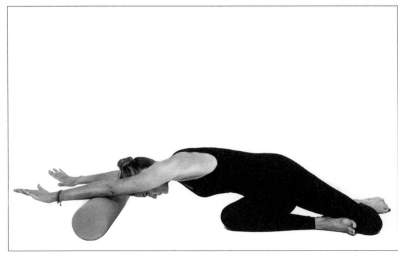

Rotating Wood Chopper

- Stand in a straddle position, with your feet about five feet apart. Hold on to either edge of the roller and reach your arms overhead.
- Inhale and begin bending to the right.
- When you have bent about halfway, rotate your torso down toward the right side of the mat. Be sure to keep your knees soft so you don't stress your back or knee joints.
- Gently swing the roller over to the left, using your waist to draw your upper body over to the left side, and then back up to stand.

Repeat this movement three times, then repeat on the other side.

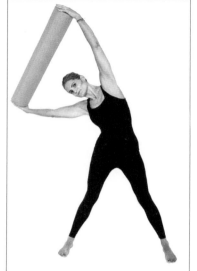
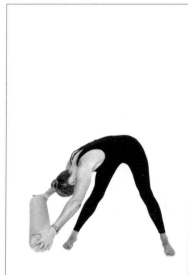
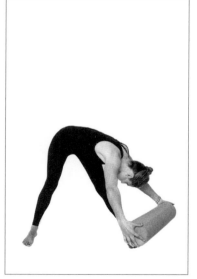
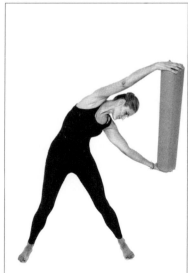

Side Kicks

- Hinge your legs at a 45-degree angle, with your heels together. Place the roller between your right lower rib cage and right hip. Bend your left elbow to bring your left hand lightly behind your head; bring your right forearm to the mat with your thumb pointing up, and your right elbow slightly behind your right shoulder.
- Inhale as you use your belly to lift your legs, maintaining your upper body posture.
- Exhale as you lower your legs, leaving them to hover slightly over the mat.

Repeat this motion ten times on each side.

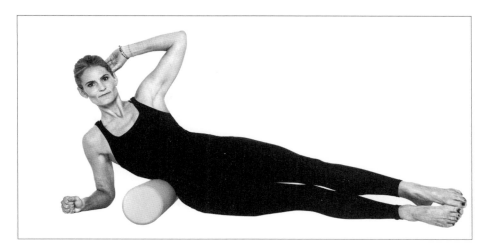

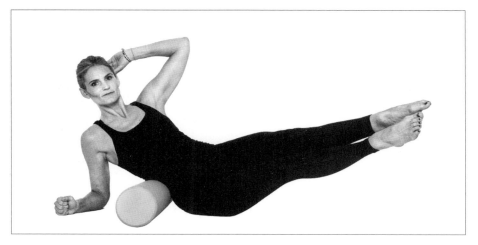

Slinky Spine

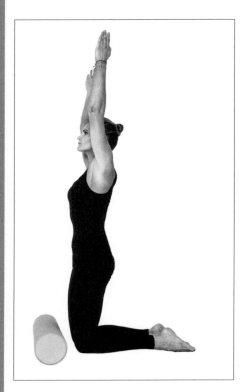

- Kneel, placing the roller a few inches in front of you. Inhale as you reach your arms up.
- Exhale as you round your spine down to roll into a kneeling forward fold that looks like an upside-down letter U. Be sure to soften your knees to help gently open the lower back.
- Inhale as you reach your spine into a full extension, chest down and sitz bones up; roll the roller up your forearms.
- Inhale to curl your tailbone under and pull your belly in as you roll yourself back up to the starting position like a Slinky.

Repeat this movement four times.

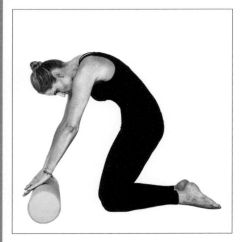

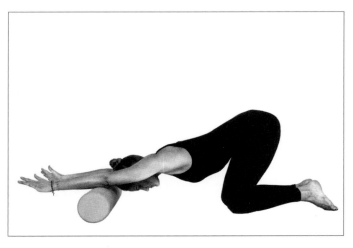

Spinal Articulation

- Place the roller under your midback at your bra line. Place your feet on the floor hip width apart, knees bent. Keep your hips heavy on the mat. Interlace your hands behind your head to support your head and neck.

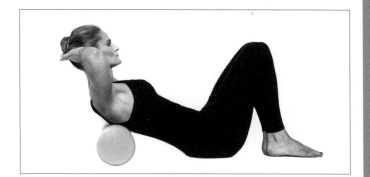

- Keeping the roller stable, inhale as you extend your upper back over the roller to mobilize your thoracic spine.
- Exhale as you curl back up.
- Next, push into your feet to move the roller up your spine one inch. Inhale as you extend and arch your back over the roller. Exhale as you curl back

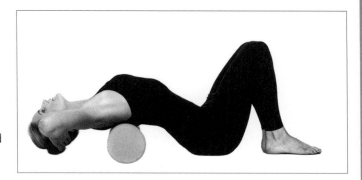

up. Keep going up your spine inch by inch until you have rolled all the way up to the top of your shoulders.
- Reverse your way back down your spine in the same manner until the roller reaches the bottom of your rib cage.

Repeat the entire process three times.

Standing Side Bends

- Stand up tall with your feet hip width apart and knees soft. With arms shoulder-width apart, hold the roller overhead.
- Inhale to reach up and over to the right to open up the left side of your body.
- Exhale to reach up and over to the left to open up the right side of your body.

Repeat this movement five times on each side, alternating sides.

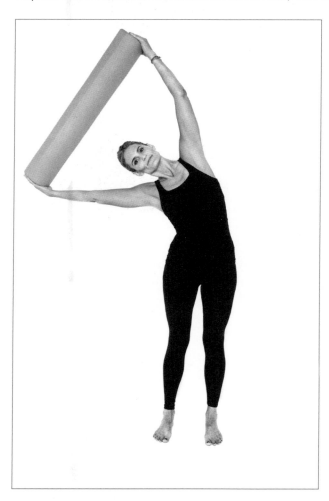

Starfish

- Come down to the mat and sit on your sitz bones. Place your right shin in front of you and your left shin out to the left side so that your knees are staggered. Place the roller to the right of you and place the palm of your right hand on the roller.
- Keeping the roller stable, lift your hips up and forward while you reach your left arm up and back, following your arm with your gaze elongating the neck.
- Inhale as you start lowering your hips back down, simultaneously curling your chin and neck back down and circling your arm in front of you toward the roller.

Repeat this movement six times, then repeat on the other side.

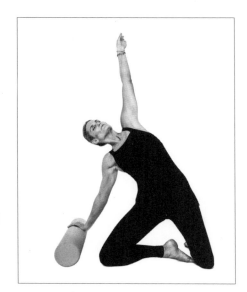

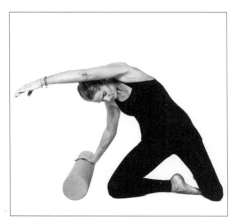

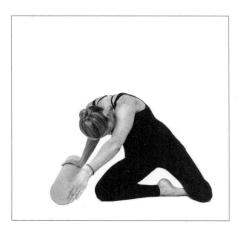

Acknowledgments

I am so grateful to the many individuals who have made this dream come to life. I am truly grateful for the opportunity to share with readers everywhere this knowledge I have spent my entire adult life pursuing. Thank you to my mentors, my clients, friends, and family for the support and guidance you've given me along the way.

Thank you for the focused guidance of Marnie Cochran, my fabulous and gifted editor, and the wonderful team at Ballantine/Random House. Thanks to Michele Promaulayko, Dave Zinczenko, and Coleen O'Shea for introducing me to the amazing and magical world of publishing and giving me the tools to share my knowledge. A huge thanks to the super-talented Nikki Van Noy for helping me put this knowledge into the right words so that I can communicate it in a simple and straightforward manner. Without these incredibly talented and generous people this book would not have come to fruition.

Thanks to my great friend and agent, Amy Stanton, and the entire Stanton & Co team for believing in me from the first moment without hesitation. Thanks also to Elise Loehan, Gwyneth Paltrow, and the whole team at Goop. Thank you Collin Stark and Jessica Stark for creating such amazing images for this guide.

Thank you to my dear and loyal clients; Kristen Miller-Langley for being my muse and Maggie Langley for being my mentor, Patricia Thirsk, Peter Nolan, Liza Rosen, Baron Davis, and Jarret Stoll for believing in me and trusting me and being my guinea pigs. I'm so grateful to you all for allowing me to be creative and develop this program with your help—and of course for allowing me to test my theories on you! I am only able to do what I do with passion and knowledge that this program truly works because of your constant support and encouragement. Thanks to Melissa Rauch and Gabby Reece for your guidance and support through this process.

Thanks to Dan, Steve and Aimee for teaching me Structural Integration at the New School of Structural Integration. Thanks to Stacy Vargas adn Sara Dacklin for inspiring me and teaching me true classical Pilates.

Thanks to my dad and Christie and the rest of my family for putting up with my ambition. I also want to acknowledge my late and much loved mother, Jean, who's brave battle with cancer that began when I was a teenager provided the motivation to spend my life exploring this path of health and wellness.

Thank you to Betty Jones for teaching me TM and helping me connect and honor my gifts.

And lastly to my beloved husband, Gus Roxburgh, and our daughter, Cameron, for believing in me and supporting me every step of the way.

ABOUT THE AUTHOR

Named one of *Shape Magazine*'s Top 50 Hottest Trainers in America in 2014, LAUREN ROXBURGH is certified in the fields of Structural Integration, Pilates, yoga, massage, meditation, and nutrition. She has an A-list client base in Los Angeles and New York, including some of the world's best orthopedic surgeons. A regular contributor to *Goop* and a member of the advisory board of Yahoo Health, she is the go-to-writer and expert for all things fascia and foam rolling.

laurenroxburgh.com